Osteoporosis & Osteopenia

Vitamin Therapy for Stronger Bones

Osteoporosis & Osteopenia

Vitamin Therapy for Stronger Bones

Bryant Lusk

Names: Lusk, Bryant, author.

Title: Osteoporosis & osteopenia: vitamin therapy for stronger bones / Bryant Lusk.

Description: First edition. | Chicago : Bryant Lusk, [2019]

Identifiers: ISBN: 978-1-7336425-0-7 (print) | 978-1-7336425-1-4 (eBook) | LCCN: 2019901533

Subjects: LCSH: Osteoporosis--Diet therapy. | Osteoporosis--Alternative treatment. | Osteopenia--Diet therapy. | Osteopenia--Alternative treatment. | Vitamin therapy. | Vitamins in human nutrition. | Dietary supplements. | Bones--Diseases--Diet therapy. | Bones--Diseases-- Nutritional aspects. | Minerals--Health aspects. | Hormones--Health aspects. | Women--Diseases--Nutritional aspects. | Men--Diseases--Nutritional aspects. | BISAC: HEALTH & FITNESS / Diseases / Musculoskeletal. | HEALTH & FITNESS / Women's Health. | HEALTH & FITNESS / Men's Health. | | HEALTH & FITNESS / Naturopathy. | MESH: Bone Density-- physiology. | Osteoporotic Fractures--prevention & control. | Vitamins--therapeutic use.

Classification: LCC: RC931.O73 L87 2019 | DDC: 616.7/1--dc23

Special discounts and permanent paper copies are available on quantity purchases. For details, visit https://bryantlusk.com/b2b/

ISBN 978-1-7336425-0-7 (paperback)
ISBN 978-1-7336425-1-4 (eBook)

LCCN 2019901533

1. Vitamins for osteoporosis prevention. 2. Low bone density treatment. 3. Bone quality. 4. Bone loss. 5. Title.

First Edition

 a PennedSource Production

Cover designed by Cherie Foxley

To Brittany Roston and her wonderful grandparents.

CONTENTS

LIST OF TABLES

Sincere Acknowledgments

The following institutions maintain much of the research used to support this work. Their members work tirelessly behind the scenes to improve the health and wellbeing of us all.

- National Institutes of Health (NIH).
- National Cancer Institute (NCI).
- National Institute of Mental Health (NIMH).
- National Library of Medicine (NLM).
- Office of Dietary Supplements (ODS).
- Centers for Disease Control and Prevention (CDC).
- World Health Organization (WHO).
- National Center for Health Statistics (NCHS).
- Food and Drug Administration (FDA).

Additionally, every medical professional and their staff deserve recognition for their momentous contributions to our health and quality of life. I thank each and every one of you.

No author produces a work they can be truly proud of without significant assistance from others. Therefore, I must highlight my small team of literary and graphics masters.

- Ann Bridges (Lead Editor)
- Cherie Foxley (Cover Design)

"Silently and without warning, bones may begin to weaken early in life if you do not have a healthy diet and the right kinds of physical activity. Many people already have weak bones and don't know it. Others are making choices that will weaken their bones later.

There are several kinds of bone disease. The most common is osteoporosis. In this disease, bones lose minerals like calcium. They become fragile and break easily. With osteoporosis, your body's frame becomes like the frame of a house damaged by termites. Termites weaken your house like osteoporosis weakens your bones. If you have severe fractures from osteoporosis, you risk never walking again. Weak bones can break easily. This can be fatal.

Fragile bones are not painful at first. Unfortunately, most people don't realize they have weakened bones until one breaks. By that time, it is hard to make your bones strong again."[1]

- The United States Surgeon General -

Introduction

Bones are in a state of constant renovation as they are stripped of old material and restored with new. This activity occurs every second of every day for your entire life. Now you can maximize your bone-building process with minimal disruption to your daily life.

As a credentialed Safety Inspector and Quality Control Specialist, I look at complex processes to find the gaps, waste, and conflicts within them. The human body's bone-building process is amazing! It uses extremely basic compounds to grow and support living tissue, which is an extraordinary feat unto itself. These and other fascinating occurrences are going on inside of us to keep our bones strong and healthy.

The information offered here provides a path of least resistance to stronger bones and a healthier life. Moreover, the strategy presented will enable you to achieve long-term results with only the smallest investments in your health. Because of my training, I am keenly aware of human factors that lead to the failure of overly burdensome routines. My goal is to share with you a simple approach toward significantly improving bone quality and overall health.

Although there are many factors involved in osteoporosis and osteopenia—such as genetics—a primary cause is the improper quantity and ratio of the vitamins and minerals that we consume. Moreover, maintaining a healthy liver is critical for achieving high bone density. Popular fat-burning products have been shown to injure the liver, which is detrimental to the bone building process. Therefore, you are going to be introduced to two searchable databases that will enable you to identify products that can damage your liver and weaken your bones.

Additionally, key factors such as direct and indirect bone nutrition knowledge, the best foods and vitamin formulations, and when to take your supplements are all discussed here. Included in the discussion are fact-based responses to the myths and misinformation regarding vitamin D, iodine, and more.

To make your life easier, daily supplementation schedules are included for different age groups. The calendars I created take into account age-related variables, such as income, lifestyles, and nutritional needs. Moreover, I go a step further by identifying several supplement options to get the best quality for cost.

I have no financial interests in the products I recommend. My only interest is in sharing information to improve your quality of life.

References to "superfoods," magic diets, and mystical secrets from faraway lands are not contained in this book. However, you will discover a sustainable, common-sense approach to building stronger bones.

When appropriately applied, vitamin therapy can transform your system into a full-time antagonist to bone loss, even while you sleep. It also delivers an array of additional health benefits, including faster healing and protection against disease. The more you read, the more you will realize the level of control at your command.

The information has not been cherry-picked to support foregone conclusions. My goal, again, is to show you a path of least resistance to superior bone quality and overall health—a path you won't mind walking for the rest of your life.

Young Adults

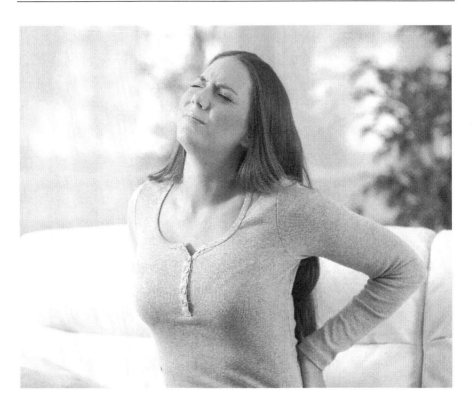

Through an internal process called bone remodeling, the average person will rebuild more than seven complete skeletons over time.[2] Younger adults can reap the greatest benefit from this life-long process. Now is the time to take full advantage of your bone-building capacity: the stronger your bones are by age thirty, the stronger they will remain throughout the rest of your life. Bone health is not a topic solely for individuals age sixty and older...it is an important and exciting subject for us all.

How to Use This Book

Osteoporosis & Osteopenia: Vitamin Therapy for Stronger Bones is structured for three types of readers: those who can never get enough information, those who just want to get to it, and those who fall somewhere in between.

If you fall somewhere in the middle, consider starting at the paragraph heading "How Much and How Often" within the chapters. Make sure to also read the "Daily Supplement Schedule" for your age group and the remaining chapters after it.

For individuals who just want to get to it, go directly to the "Daily Supplement Schedule" for your age group. You will find the schedules to be straightforward. You are encouraged to refer to the paragraph headings "How Much and How Often" in each of the previous chapters.

Avid consumers of information should start at the very beginning of each chapter. I have tried not to overburden you while still providing enough information to quench your thirst for knowledge.

A preferred list of vitamin and mineral products is included with the *Daily Supplement Schedules*.

CHAPTER ONE

Life Expectancy

According to the International Osteoporosis Foundation, just under nine million fractures a year are attributed to osteoporosis.[3,4] Osteoporosis is an extremely debilitating ailment whose onset occurs too frequently and too rapidly in many individuals. Osteopenia (decreased bone density) is viewed as the precursor to osteoporosis. If you currently suffer from osteoporosis, osteopenia, or poor bone quality, the progression of these ailments can be addressed and your condition can improve. However, before we get into the meat of the subject, we need to talk a bit about longevity.

As with many aspects of the human condition, age directly impacts our bone health. The longer you live, the more disciplined you need to be to prevent low bone density and reduced bone quality from affecting your life. Average life expectancy has increased dramatically over the last century, from just forty-nine years at the turn of the twentieth century to over seventy-six years by 1996. By 2008, white females (of Hispanic and non-Hispanic origin) maintained the highest life expectancy in the United States at 80.9 years, followed by black females at 77.2 years.[5]

On average, people in their twenties today will live well into their nineties and possibly low one hundreds. Healthy bone structure is vital to their future.

Although there is no magic bullet for optimum health, one undeniable fact is that many people lack adequate levels of the vitamins and minerals their cells need for maximum fitness, performance, and appearance. This is especially true regarding bone health. Vitamins and minerals supply the energy and materials you need to develop and maintain strong, healthy bones. The amounts and ratios of these nutrients are vital. Too much of any critical substance, such as phosphorous, can be just as devastating to your bone health as too little. Therefore, our goal is to strike the right balance.

Your Miraculous Bones

Bones are far more incredible than most people realize. They continually reform and rebuild themselves throughout your life. Without bones, we would either have exoskeletons (like spiders) or be masses of formless tissue, slithering our way through life. Instead, we can stand tall, build massive structures, enjoy numerous activities, and give powerful hugs to those we love.

In fact, bones maintain our internal pH balance by releasing calcium into our bloodstream when needed. This tightly regulated process is vital to our very existence. If this process were to ever stop working within an individual, that person would die in a manner of seconds. Our bones also serve as our protectors by shielding our lungs, heart, spinal cord, and brain. These are only a few of the many reasons we need to protect and nourish our bones. Hormones also play a big role in bone production. After a few chapters, we are going to begin identifying simple solutions to frequently overlooked conditions in order to optimize your bone-building capability.

The following images are three-dimensional renderings of human bone. They depict stages of progression of osteoporosis from left (normal bone) to right (osteoporosis). The image on the far left displays higher bone density than the one on the far right.

Figure 1. Osteoporosis Progression

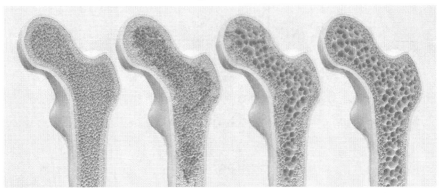

The bone structure on the right is likely more susceptible to curvature and fractures due to the lower density. However, a person with low bone density can still have an adequate level of bone "quality," making them resistant to fractures and injury. Also, a person can have a suitable level of bone density, yet poor bone quality, making them susceptible to fractures and injury.

Osteopenia is defined as having lower than normal bone density, but not so low as to cross the threshold into osteoporosis. However, if left untreated, osteopenia can develop into osteoporosis over time. Osteopenia occurs (relatively) at or just after the second bone structure depicted in the image.

Condition-Based Risk Factors

The following conditions moderately or significantly increase the risk of developing osteoporosis. Some are due to the condition itself; others are due to medications such as prednisone, cortisone, and corticosteroids administered as a result of the condition.[6]

- Alcoholism
- Anorexia nervosa
- Asthma
- Bed rest and immobilization
- Breast cancer
- Celiac disease
- Diabetes (Type 1)
- Gastric Bypass Surgery
- Inflammatory bowel disease
- Lactose intolerance
- Lupus
- Nonalcoholic Fatty Liver Disease (NAFLD)
- Osteogenesis imperfecta
- Prostate cancer
- Rheumatoid arthritis
- Smoking

Minerals, Tests, and Misinformation

Bones are living tissue comprised mostly of minerals and collagen. The cells that build these powerful structures require a steady supply of specific hormones and minerals to maintain their structure. Mineral deficiencies are one of the greatest obstacles to building and maintaining strong bones. Unfortunately, standard blood tests for certain mineral levels are incredibly unreliable. Magnesium is one example.[7,8,9]

Just over 50 percent of the magnesium in your body is stored inside of your bones. Slightly less than 50 percent resides in your muscle and soft tissue. Less than 1 percent of your magnesium is contained in your blood. That minuscule amount often fluctuates due to everyday activities, such as a stressful day at work. Because of these and other reasons, blood tests conducted to determine magnesium levels are not reliable.

Table 1. Measured Magnesium in Adults[10]

Blood Serum + RBC	0.8 percent
Muscle + Soft Tissue	46.3 percent
Bone	52.9 percent

A magnesium deficiency will commonly manifest itself as muscle cramps, muscle twitches, fatigue, heart palpitations, and even cardiac arrhythmia.[11,12,13] In fact, these and other symptoms are common triggers for mineral blood tests. My blood tested negative for mineral deficiencies even after displaying severe muscle cramping and an unusual heartbeat. My symptoms ended within days of adding supplemental potassium and magnesium to my diet.

A person would have to be severely deficient to consistently test positive for low magnesium levels in their blood serum. The bone-building process will be compromised during the time it takes to become chronically magnesium deficient.

When it comes to serious, debilitating ailments, you would be far better served by an early warning system that delivers accurate results. Seven years ago, after combing through mountains of research at home and abroad, I found a doctor in the USA who developed a more precise testing method.

The technical term for the procedure is "sublingual epithelial cell analysis."[14,15] This method of testing should be considered for several reasons, accuracy being chief among them. The method used to collect the cells for this procedure is virtually painless. It requires your doctor to secure a sample of your cells via a mouth swab, similar to collecting a DNA sample. The doctor sends your sample to a lab that uses analytical scanning electron microscopy (ASEM) and elemental X-ray analysis (EXA) to measure the mineral content inside your cells.

More importantly, the results are so accurate, they are used to evaluate the ratio between mineral electrolytes within your cells. The following minerals are tested: magnesium, calcium, potassium, phosphorus, sodium, and chloride. Knowing that a doctor of your choosing is involved in the process increases my confidence in this procedure.

The cost for this test is just over three hundred dollars at the time that I became aware of it. Prices are subject to change. Your insurance provider may cover a portion of the expenses associated with the evaluation. Additionally, a percentage of the cost may be covered by Medicare. More information on how to request this test, what they test for, and the lab that conducts it can be found online at www.exatest.com.

Blood tests do provide extremely useful information and are a powerful diagnostic tool. However, when it comes to the real danger of mineral deficiencies impeding bone-building productivity, the information they provide is unreliable.

Bone-Building Process

Bones are high-maintenance items. In basic terms, they require a 24/7 demolition crew, a 24/7 team of builders, and a continuous supply of raw materials. Hormones run the factory. Low bone density occurs when your internal bone demolition crew outperforms your bone building crew over an extended period (typically years). There are various reasons this condition occurs, such as genetics, lifestyle, diet, age, and medications.

The bone demolition crew within us is made up of millions of cells called **osteoclasts** (clasts with a "c"). Osteoclasts are constantly strip-mining your bones of old material to make room for new material. Think of it as removing old wood from a door frame to replace it with fresh wood.

The bone building crew that installs fresh bone material is made up of millions of cells called **osteoblasts** (blasts with a "b"). Osteoblasts require a few items to do their job properly: they need raw material for new bone, and they also need a substance to bind (infuse) new bone onto your existing structure. That binding agent is an extremely specialized protein called **osteocalcin**.[16,17] Although there are more cellular processes directly involved, these are the three we will explore.

Hormones such as estrogen, testosterone, progesterone, calcitriol (vitamin D), and parathyroid are the primary factors in your body's creation and utilization of osteoclasts (demolition cells), osteoblasts (building cells), and osteocalcin (the bone material binding agent). Vitamin and hormone deficiencies diminish osteoblasts production and increase osteoclasts activity, resulting in accelerated bone deterioration as indicated in the following figure.

Figure 2. Bone Growth and Loss Projections

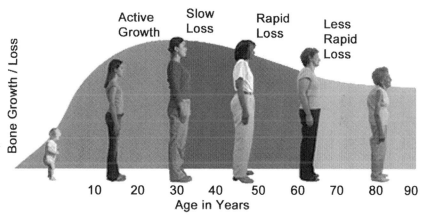

1[Untitled image of osteoporosis progression]. Retrieved January 26, 2019, https://www.bones.nih.gov/health-info/bone/SGR/surgeon-generals-report

Fortunately, no one is destined to have their bones decline in this manner. To that end, I have identified specific vitamins and minerals your bones need for optimal health. I will also introduce vitamin and mineral cofactors, which are often ignored, yet impact bone health in multiple ways.

We constantly need to create and stimulate osteoblasts to match or outperform the work of their demolition cell counterparts. Osteoblasts cells create osteocalcin, which is another reason we need to support their productivity.

Any impediment or disruption of your bone-building process will result in less-than-optimal bone health. Osteoporosis does not occur overnight. It is a condition that gradually develops over several years. It is never too late for anyone to take measures that will slow, stop, or even reverse the progress of this ailment.

Men and women are both affected by osteoporosis. In the United States, more than forty million people already have osteoporosis, or are at high risk of developing it. What statistics often overlook is the impact on the loved ones of those who suffer from this condition. They too will benefit by learning and sharing the information in this book.

Bone Density Test

A dual-energy X-ray absorptiometry (DXA) scan is conducted to determine bone density. Specialized equipment measures your hip, spine, and, at times, your entire skeletal structure. Upon completion, your bone density is rated with a T-score.

Table 2. Bone Density T-Score Chart

+1 to -1 indicates normal bone mass.
-1 to -2.5 indicates low bone mass (osteopenia).
-2.5 and lower indicates you have osteoporosis.

Medicare Part B covers this test once every twenty-four months, or more often under certain conditions.

There is also a Z-score, which is derived from the difference between measured bone density and the anticipated density for your age, ethnicity, gender, and weight. Quantitative computed tomography (QCT) is another bone imaging technique.

Bone scanning procedures are initially performed on individuals age 65 and older unless there is an underlying condition. However, nothing prevents you from getting a bone health evaluation at any age. You might consider requesting a baseline-scan between the ages of 25–40, followed by additional scans every five to ten years. Results between different equipment may vary. Always consult with your doctor.

Trabecular Bone Score (TBS)–Bone Quality Test

Bone density is one indicator of bone health. Trabecular bone quality is also a significant factor. In general, the human skeleton is made up of approximately 20 percent trabecular bone and 80 percent cortical bone.[18]

These percentages differ within the various sections of bone inside of your body. For instance, the human vertebra (spine) is comprised, largely, of trabecular bone. Vertebra suffer the highest rate of fracture in individuals with osteoporosis. Over time, vertebral fractures can cause chronic back pain and curvature of the spine.

Some time ago, medical and scientific communities began to notice that individuals who do not have osteoporosis still make up a sizeable percentage of hip fracture occurrences. Additionally, many individuals with osteoporosis never suffered a fracture. As they studied this phenomenon more closely, it was determined that regardless of bone density, trabecular bone quality is integral to the overall health and resilience of bone tissue. Even if you have low bone density, good bone quality can prevent fractures and mitigate bone injury.

Trabecular bone score (TBS) data is generated by high resolution peripheral quantitative computed tomography (HRpQCT), an imaging process that measures and correlates bone texture with bone microarchitecture.[19,20,21] Basically, it provides imaging data to assess the structural integrity of your bone material. TBS technology has been developed by companies such as Medimaps Group, a Swiss company, and QUIBIM S.L., a company based in Spain with at least one office in Palo Alto, California.

Osteoporosis (Good News)

For many people, preventing osteoporosis and improving bone quality is very feasible. Additionally, individuals who have already succumbed to this condition can rebound from it and improve their quality of life. Remember, the stronger you can make your bones by the time you hit your early thirties, the stronger they will remain throughout the rest of your life.

Physical activity is important for building and maintaining strong bones. However, many individuals find it challenging to follow a rigid exercise regime. Unless you intend to work yourself into a chiseled masterpiece, a few dumbbells and resistance bands will do just fine. If you currently have osteoporosis, sudden-impact exercise maneuvers that exert a high level of force on your bones should be avoided.

Whether you decide to exercise or not, there is nothing preventing you from taking a few vitamins each day. I encourage you to think in terms of amplification: even the slightest input can yield major results. You do not have to choose between doing everything that is good for your bones, or nothing at all.

Consider individuals who do not exercise and have a less-than-healthy diet. Although I encourage these individuals to improve their diet and to quit bad habits, they can still improve their bone health simply by taking certain high-yield vitamins and minerals. Do not succumb to the erroneous ideology of "all or nothing." Rather, think in terms of degrees. Anything you do to improve your bone health is better than doing nothing at all.

The challenge is knowing which vitamins to take, which brands to trust, and how often to take them—you overcame every part of this challenge when you purchased this book. Knowing the limits before a vitamin becomes hazardous is also discussed here. The investment you have made by purchasing this book can truly impact the rest of your life.

Hand-Picked Vitamins and Minerals

Many dynamics influence the health and strength of our bones such as hormones, age, activity level, and genetics. The simplest and most manageable factor at your fingertips is vitamin therapy, which can dramatically improve your bone, liver, and hormone productivity.

There are numerous benefits to be gained from vitamin therapy. Vitamins and minerals that strengthen bones also reduce the risk of developing a multitude of chronic health problems, including hypertension and heart disease.

Some vitamin advocates recommend massive amounts of certain nutrients to achieve specific outcomes. They discuss individual vitamins and minerals from a singular perspective, versus as part of an overall system.

My philosophy represents the polar opposite. Nutrients and hormones are synergetic. I liken them to a world-class symphony, in which every instrument and note must work in concert to deliver the best performance. Vitamins and minerals are more effective when they are in balance. Flooding your system with a single substance can cause an imbalance, resulting in more harm than good. I urge you not to follow the latest, greatest vitamin fad. More isn't better—balance is. I explain my views on this quite extensively throughout the book.

Getting Started

Regarding vitamin therapy, my first suggestion is to stop purchasing vitamins from the average grocery or drugstore. There are a few, basic vitamins that may work well regardless of the manufacturer. However, when considering your health and quality of life, you are encouraged to invest in vitamin products seldom found in your local grocery store (with few exceptions).

Instead, purchase your products from an actual vitamin store or directly from the manufacturer's website. This is where you will find vitamins and minerals with a significantly higher level of quality. I have provided several options of manufacturers and products for you to choose from throughout the book. However, as mentioned earlier, you will find a complete list in the chapter, *Daily Supplement Schedules*.

My second suggestion is to be vigilant when purchasing vitamins through third-party internet retailers. One is especially known for offering free two-day shipping. The problem is not with the retailer; rather, there are issues with some of the sellers who market to consumers through them. There have been instances of sellers shipping counterfeit or expired products. This does not happen often, but it does happen frequently enough to warrant concern.

If you choose to purchase online through third-party retailers, read the reviews for the seller. Examine the product and be sure to read the expiration date. Some sellers have even stooped to covering expiration dates with barcode labels. Do not become frightened or overly cautious, but do be careful.

Now that you've learned a bit about bone structure and the bone-building process, let's continue by focusing on a remarkable mineral that is easy to obtain. I began telling friends and colleagues about this underrated substance nearly a decade ago. Today, it is quickly becoming the talk of the town. This basic substance supports our physiology in many ways. Correcting a deficiency in this mineral can literally change your life.

CHAPTER FOUR

Magnesium

Impacts: Bone Health, Blood Pressure, Heart Health, Weight Loss, Depression, Muscle Cramps, Menstrual Cramps, Diabetes, Protein Synthesis, Migraines, Sleep Disorders, Fatigue, ADHD, Kidney Stones, Nervous System, Cancer

Previously, I discussed magnesium in terms of mineral testing. Now I will detail the multitude of benefits this single mineral has in store for you.

Magnesium is one of your most powerful allies against low bone density and poor bone quality. Adequate levels are required for anyone who seeks to optimize bone health. Unfortunately, magnesium is severely lacking in the typical diet, and magnesium deficiency is quickly becoming a global issue. Bones are made up primarily of calcium, phosphorous, collagen, and—to a lesser extent—magnesium. Do not let the "lesser extent" fool you: magnesium plays a substantial role in the health and structure of your bones.[22,23]

Vitamin manufacturers are beginning to appreciate the magnesium/vitamin D connection. In a nutshell, the vitamin D you consume or develop from sun exposure does absolutely nothing for you. It floats about in your system in a dormant state until it is transformed: first into 25-hydroxyvitamin D, and then into an active hormone, **calcitriol** $(1,25(OH)2D)$.

Calcitriol does numerous things for you and plays a significant role in the absorption and utilization of calcium and phosphate. These elements are critical for the healthy structure and remodeling of your bones. Calcitriol is essential to the creation of osteoblasts as it transfers DNA coding into new cells in order to create more of them. The more osteoblasts you have, the stronger your bones will be.

Magnesium is the catalyst that enables you to effectively transform vitamin D3 from its dormant state into the active hormone that your bone-building factory so desperately needs. We will discuss this in more detail in Chapter 7 on vitamin D.

Without magnesium, your bone-building factory would grind to a halt. However, your heart would completely seize before that happened. Moreover, more than three hundred processes that work to keep you alive and healthy require magnesium. Adequate (not excessive) magnesium intake is a common missing link to stronger bones and better health.

Recall that osteoblasts are the cells that literally build your bones every second of every day throughout your life. Osteoblast population growth is impeded by low magnesium levels, resulting in fewer bone construction cells.[24] Moreover, low magnesium increases your number of bone demolition cells (osteoclasts).[25] You need the proper balance of both for healthy bones. Women with osteoporosis have been shown to have lower magnesium levels than women who do not suffer from this ailment.[26, 27]

Magnesium is necessary for many metabolic functions, including DNA synthesis, protein synthesis, and neurotransmission. Studies identify magnesium deficiency as a risk factor for various forms of cancer, including breast cancer.[28,29] In addition, magnesium is beneficial for weight-loss.[30]

Magnesium deficiency also appears to be linked to depression. According to one study, "a variety of neuromuscular and psychiatric symptoms, including different types of depression, was observed in magnesium deficiency."[31] In another study, participants with lower magnesium intake reported higher levels of depression.[32]

As vital as magnesium is to your mental and physical health, magnesium deficiency is all too common in the United States and abroad. This is especially true among African Americans and the elderly.

How Much and How Often

It is very challenging to obtain adequate amounts of magnesium through food and drink alone. Foods containing the highest concentrations, such as almonds and spinach, provide only about 20 percent of the recommended daily allowance (RDA) per serving.

Given the average American diet, many people may have to supplement at least 75 percent of their daily magnesium requirement to maintain adequate levels. The need for supplementation increases with high-intensity activities and age.

The RDA for magnesium is 310–320 mg (for women) and 400–420 mg (for men). Based on the tolerable upper intake level (UL), if you take 350 mg (or more) at one time, you may develop an upset stomach and diarrhea.

The average person can only absorb up to 180 mg of magnesium per dose. Of course, everyone is a little different, but this is the general rule. For example, I take 266–399 mg of magnesium glycinate every day. I accomplish this by taking one 133 mg capsule (or tablet) two or three times per day with meals, or one 200 mg tablet twice per day with meals. It took all of two days for me to notice significant results. Among other things, muscle cramps and a sudden-onset irregular heartbeat became a thing of the past.

If you are magnesium deficient, you should notice results within days, including but not limited to fewer muscle cramps, diminished menstrual cramps, and deeper sleep. Long-term effects often include improved heart function, improved blood pressure, better insulin regulation, stronger bones and teeth, and improved mineral utilization. Vitamin D levels and utilization should also improve.

You do not need excessive doses to achieve results. Balance is a primary factor for optimal mental and physical health.

Table 3. Magnesium–Food

Food Type and Quantity	How Often
pumpkin seeds, 1 ounce. almonds, dry roasted, 1 ounce. spinach, boiled, ½ cup. swiss chard, 1 cup. cashews, dry roasted, 1 ounce. peanuts, oil roasted, ¼ cup. black beans, cooked, ½ cup. peanut butter, 2 tablespoons. bread, whole wheat, 2 slices. avocado, cubed, 1 cup.	One serving of any of these food items, 5 to 8 times a day, 5 to 7 days per week. Always consider calories and fat intake.

Table 4. Magnesium–Supplement

Suggested Supplement Options	How Much and How Often
Swanson – Chelated Magnesium Bisglycinate (133 mg). Whole Foods 365 – Magnesium Glycinate (~133 mg). Now Foods – Magnesium Citrate (200 mg). Good State – Ionic (liquid) Magnesium (100 mg). Doctor's Best – Chelated Magnesium Glycinate (100 mg).	200-400 mg 5 to 7 days per week. Or a combination of foods (listed above) and supplements. For maximum absorption do not exceed 200 mg in a single dose. Do not take with calcium.

Absorption Inhibitors

Calcium strongly inhibits the absorption of magnesium. Therefore, I do not recommend supplements that combine magnesium with calcium. Foods high in phytates or oxalates such as grains, bran, unsprouted beans, soy, spinach, leafy greens, and nuts inhibit magnesium absorption to some degree. Do not be overly concerned—you will still absorb some magnesium with these foods, just not the maximum amount. Alcoholic beverages, soda, stress, bleached sugar, intense workouts, and diabetes deplete the body's magnesium stores.

Absorption Enhancers

Vitamin D enhances magnesium absorption. Complex carbohydrates, protein (other than soy), and medium-chain triglycerides (MCTs), such as coconut oil and palm oil, strengthen the intake of magnesium.

A quality formulation such as magnesium-bisglycinate, made by a reputable manufacturer, will absorb extremely well. Taking two or three smaller doses will enable you to absorb more magnesium than taking one large dose.

Best Formulation

- Magnesium Glycinate (calming, relaxant effect that may aid sleep).
- Magnesium Citrate.
- Magnesium Aspartate.
- Magnesium Taurate.
- Ionic (liquid) Magnesium.

The formulations (above) are absorbed well. In contrast, the absorption rate of magnesium oxide is extremely low: approximately 4 percent. You will find that many popular multivitamin brands contain magnesium oxide—always check the nutrition label.

I commonly take Swanson Chelated Magnesium Bisglycinate (small capsules), KAL Magnesium Glycinate (The Vitamin Shoppe), and Whole Foods' 365 Magnesium Glycinate (sold at convenient locations). Always read the nutrition label when purchasing supplements.

Formulations to Avoid

The following formulations should be avoided. They are not harmful to you, but offer diminished returns on your investment because they do not absorb well.

- Magnesium oxide – Abysmal absorption rate. Very cheap to manufacture, which is why you will find it in several locations and formulations.

- Magnesium complex – Here is where manufacturers often pull a fast one. Read the ingredients. If magnesium oxide is one of the elements, do not purchase. The label will often read "magnesium glycinate, magnesium aspartate, magnesium oxide." However, it often does not stipulate the percentage of each type. Assume the majority of the product is comprised of magnesium oxide.

- Calcium with magnesium – It is possible that manufacturers believe magnesium aids in the absorption of calcium inside your gut. Magnesium does in fact aid in the absorption of calcium. However, as we just discussed, this is achieved primarily by magnesium supporting the conversion process of vitamin D3 to the active hormone [1,25(OH)2 D] calcitriol. This conversion occurs inside your liver and kidneys, not inside of your gut. In fact, calcium prevents magnesium absorption inside your gut to a large extent. If your goal is to absorb magnesium, you do not want to mix calcium with magnesium. You will still absorb some, but not nearly as much as you would without including calcium. Protein may counter the effect of calcium's interference with magnesium absorption, to some extent.

Listen to Your Body

Symptoms of magnesium deficiency include depression, anxiety, hypertension, muscle cramps, muscle knots, bone disorders, sensations of numbness or tingling, irregular heartbeat, loss of appetite, nausea, fatigue, sleep disorders, severe menstrual cramps, seizures, memory lapses, hallucinations, and disorientation.

You will probably not suffer all these things at once. However, if you suffer from any one or a combination of these symptoms, they may be caused or exacerbated by low magnesium. If you choose to supplement, do not go overboard.

Warning

Typical effects of excessive magnesium intake include diarrhea and abdominal cramping.

Testing

In many instances, blood tests can reveal a lot about your health. However, as discussed earlier, measuring blood serum magnesium levels is an incredibly unreliable way to identify a deficiency.

The average person will probably display a variety of symptoms resulting from long-term magnesium deficiency. These symptoms could include frequent muscle spasms, heart arrhythmia, or even osteoporosis. Again, blood serum tests are typically used to verify a magnesium deficiency AFTER the onset of symptoms.

Soft tissue is apparently a better test candidate for determining magnesium levels inside your body. Testing soft tissue is reportedly far more accurate for determining mineral content in the human body than testing blood serum levels. The previously discussed sublingual epithelial cell analysis (EXA test) can be initiated via www.exatest.com.

Methods for identifying a potential deficiency include:

- Recognizing symptoms (ref: *Listen to Your Body*)
- Sublingual epithelial cell analysis (EXA test).
- RBC red blood cell (this is more accurate than blood serum level).
- Diet assessment.

- Urine excretion test.
- Trial supplementation (try 200–400 mg a day and note any changes).

You are encouraged to perform additional research and to consult with your physician before subjecting yourself to any procedure.

Vitamin K2

Impacts: Bone Health, Heart Disease, Bone Disease, Arthritis, Cancer, Kidney Stones, and Tooth Decay

Vitamin K2 (a subcomponent of vitamin K) is another critical agent for maintaining healthy bones, teeth, and arteries. Consuming just 100 mcg of this incredible nutrient per day can reduce the calcium in your arteries (where you don't want it) while infusing calcium into your bones and teeth (where you do want it). Simply put, K2 prevents both calcification (hardening) of the arteries and weakening of bones.

One of the most challenging aspects of taking this supplement is that, unlike zinc and magnesium, you will not feel any rapid results. In time, you may wonder if taking K2 is a waste of effort and money. I assure you it is not. Have faith that taking vitamin K2 will yield extraordinary benefits and can extend your natural life. This fact is rooted in numerous studies conducted in several countries. Just because you don't feel a difference, doesn't mean it is not working.

Osteoblasts produce the "superglue" protein osteocalcin, which binds calcium to your bone tissue. Vitamin K2 increases bone quality and bone density by activating the osteocalcin protein.[33,34]

In one study, postmenopausal women were given vitamin K2 in its natural form of MK-7 over a three-year period. MK-7 reduced age-related decreases in bone mineral density (BMD).[35] In addition, MK-7 aided bone strength and significantly decreased the reduction of height (shrinkage) in the participants' vertebrae. Vitamin K2's ability to produce stronger bones is not speculation. It is a peer-reviewed, scientifically proven fact. An added benefit of this process is stronger teeth with potentially fewer cavities.

Vitamin K2 also reduces a common form of heart disease by activating another protein called matrix Gla protein (MGP).[36,37] This protein works by preventing calcium from building up inside the internal lining of your arteries. Therefore, the "pipes" in which blood flows to and from your heart will not clog as easily. A three-year study published in 2015 concluded that "long-term use of MK-7 supplements improves (reduces) arterial stiffness in healthy postmenopausal women."[38]

Vegetarians

Vegans and vegetarians are at greater risk of developing a K2 deficiency. Fortunately, vitamin K2 is available as a supplement.

How Much and How Often

Two available supplemental forms—MK-4 and MK-7—perform the same function. However, supplemental MK-4 is synthetic and dissipates from your blood serum within eight hours, whereas MK-7 remains in your blood serum for up to three days. It also takes significantly higher doses of MK-4 to achieve similar results obtained through relatively low doses of MK-7. Moreover, MK-7 is more readily available online and at your local vitamin store. For these reasons, I view MK-7 as the better option for supplementation.

The total daily adequate intake (AI) for naturally occurring K2 is 90 mcg (micrograms) for women and 120 mcg for men. Studies concluded that higher intake of K2 resulted in lower mortality rates.[39] I do not endorse exceeding 250 mcg MK-7 or 5 mg of MK-4 in supplemental form per day unless directed to do so by a healthcare professional. Moreover, it is perfectly fine to miss a day or two of MK-7 supplementation since a single dose remains active in your system for up to three days. You do not require very much vitamin K2 for optimal bone and cardiovascular health. Don't abuse it.

Here's a tip: it is difficult for individuals to determine the effectiveness of K2 supplementation. Rather than placing faith in one manufacturer, you might consider taking two different reputable brands. Either take them both daily or alternate between them every other day or week. If this is a bit confusing, it is perfectly fine to stick with a single brand you really trust. Just make sure it is a reputable one. Always remember: popular does not necessarily equate to reputable.

Table 5. Vitamin K2–Food

Food Type and Quantity	How Often
Natto (fermented soybeans). Head cheese. Soft cheese. Egg yolks. Chicken breasts. Chicken livers.	One serving of any of these food items, once or twice per day, four to seven days per week. Always consider calories and fat intake.

Table 6. Vitamin K2–Supplement

Suggested Supplement Options	How Much and How Often
Jarrow Formulas–MK-7 (90 mcg). Sports Research–MK-7 (100 mcg). Nutrigold–MK-7 (100 mcg). Now Foods–MK-7 (100 mcg).	90-200 mcg (micrograms) four to six days per week. Or a combination of foods (listed above) and supplements.

Absorption Inhibitors

K2 is a sub-component of K. Broad-spectrum antibiotics and medications used to lower cholesterol interfere with vitamin K. Excess vitamin A also inhibits the absorption of vitamin K.

Absorption Enhancers

Vitamin K2 is a fat-soluble nutrient. Taking a K2 supplement with a fatty meal may improve its absorption. Foods with healthy fats such as eggs (cage-free), flaxseed (oil or milled), avocados, olive oil, lake herring, lake trout, mackerel, wild salmon, sardines, and tuna are a few options to consider.

Best Formulation

- MK-7

Listen to Your Body

More research is needed to identify early symptoms of vitamin K2 deficiency and excess.

Low bone density or teeth that are soft or easily fractured may be an indication of inadequate levels of K2. The challenge is that other nutrient shortfalls may also cause the same symptoms.

Warning

If you are taking blood-thinning medications such as Warfarin, do not take vitamin K supplements without consulting with your physician. Taking vitamin D and calcium supplements without having adequate levels of K2 may increase your rate of arterial calcification. Balanced ratios are what your cells need to flourish.

Testing

The importance of this nutrient has only recently come into the nutritional spotlight. Therefore, it may be some time before reliable, verifiable testing methods are developed to measure K2 levels in individuals. Testing overall vitamin K levels may not suffice.

Very little vitamin K is stored in the body, making direct measurement rather difficult. It has been suggested that a vitamin K2 assay test may be worth considering. This test measures undercarboxylated osteocalcin as a functional marker of vitamin K2 levels. As discussed earlier, osteocalcin is the bone binding protein that is activated by the presence of vitamin K2.

Perform additional research and consult with your physician before subjecting yourself to this or any other tests. Several unreliable sources of information containing unproven scientific claims are hidden behind very impressive websites...proceed with caution.

Due to K2's impact on arterial calcification, you may also consider a coronary calcium scan, which may provide some indication regarding the effectiveness of your chosen brand of K2 supplements.

According to the National Heart, Lung, and Blood Institute (NHLBI), the coronary calcium scan looks for specks of calcium in the walls of the coronary (heart) arteries. Calcifications in the coronary arteries are an early sign of coronary heart disease (CHD). As previously mentioned, K2 activates MGP (protein), which traps and removes calcium from your arteries. Therefore, a coronary calcium scan may provide some indication as to the effectiveness of the brand that is used.

CHAPTER SIX

Zinc

Impacts: Progesterone, Bone Health, Thyroid Function, Weight Loss, Hair Health, Cholesterol, Immune System, Libido, Depression, Healing, Seizures, Asthma, ADHD, Macular Degeneration, Acne

So far, I have discussed two vital nutrients that directly impact bone density and structure. Zinc is yet another crucial mineral that supports skeletal health, thereby reducing the potential for developing osteoporosis. Unfortunately, many individuals view zinc strictly as a common cold remedy, but you will be amazed at the multitude of measurable benefits adequate (not excessive) levels of zinc can provide. For instance, maintaining appropriate zinc levels has been found to prevent bone loss and increase bone mass.[40] Zinc is also an important cofactor in vitamin D absorption, which is a major component of your bone building process.

Many individuals—especially those over the age of forty—are zinc deficient to some degree. Even a mild deficiency can have a significant impact on many aspects of your health.

As discussed in Chapter 2, osteoblasts are cells specifically tasked with building and hardening bone tissue. Zinc stimulates bone construction and mineralization by increasing osteoblast formation and activity. Zinc also reduces osteoclast (bone demolition cells) population growth. You need both osteoblast and osteoclast cells for healthy bone formation. However, a proper ratio between these cells must be maintained for optimum bone health. Zinc and magnesium are both significant factors in sustaining that ratio.

Furthermore, zinc deficiency lowers testosterone. Age-related testosterone deficiency has been viewed as the most important factor of bone loss in elderly men.[41,42] As we develop our understanding of how zinc, K2, and magnesium support the bone-building process, we also develop our roadmap to building stronger bones.

To recap, zinc directly impacts vitamin D absorption, osteoblast production, and testosterone production. Vitamin K2 activates osteocalcin, the protein needed to bind new material to your bones. It also removes calcium from the inner lining of coronary arteries. Magnesium is needed for vitamin D conversion, osteoblast production, and associated processes. Magnesium also amplifies potassium utilization and improves heart function.

Checkpoint

(resolving magnesium deficiency) + (resolving K2 deficiency) + (resolving zinc deficiency)

- leads to -

stronger and denser bone-building capability + improved immune response, testosterone levels, healing, heart function, sleep, and more...

End Checkpoint

As stated in the introduction, this simple approach is not rooted in speculation, super-foods, or wonder diets. Information has not been cherry-picked to support foregone conclusions. Everything presented thus far is rooted in peer-reviewed science. More importantly, the methods outlined are things that almost anyone can do to achieve remarkable results for their bone health. We have more ground to cover. However, it is important to ensure that we construct our roadmap along the way.

An added benefit of resolving a zinc deficiency is the nearly instantaneous relief from some forms of erectile dysfunction. Just 15 mg of high-quality zinc taken with the last meal of the day will yield amazing results for some individuals suffering from erectile dysfunction. Men in their forties and beyond will wake up like teenagers again. This will of course not work for everyone. It will, however, work in many cases. To a lesser extent, women may also notice something different in their libido within a week or two of taking zinc supplements.

Zinc plays a critical role in maintaining your immune system, along with your metabolism, thyroid health, mood, ability to heal, and more. Overall zinc levels decline as we age, compromising immune function.[43] Low zinc levels have also been linked to diabetes.[44] In turn, these functions directly affect your weight, blood pressure, energy, and sex drive. All of this plays a direct or indirect role in bone health.

Retinal zinc concentrations decline as we age, which may affect eye health. The human brain contains the highest amount of zinc. Studies show blood serum zinc levels to be low in people suffering from depression.[45] In addition, the intensity of depression appears to correlate with the degree of zinc deficiency. Depression can have a secondary effect on bone density, stemming from a lack of motivation and energy.

Zinc imbalance can also result in heightened aggression or violence. Elevated levels of copper can result from a zinc deficiency, triggering neurological disorders. In addition, a lack of zinc can contribute to neuronal injury or death.

Remarkably, a thirty-day supplementation of zinc gluconate resulted in a notable reduction in weight and BMI indices according to a 2013 research article in the Advanced Pharmaceutical Bulletin.[46] Zinc is an incredible substance that goes far beyond impeding the common cold. We are now beginning to realize how a few vitamins and minerals can literally alter the course of one's life, and even extend it. Maintaining proper zinc levels improves bone quality, lowers risk factors for additional health issues, and can improve the quality of one's life.

Vegetarians

The bioavailability (rate of absorption) of zinc from vegetarian diets is lower than from non-vegetarian foods.[47] Zinc contained in meat absorbs exceptionally well. In addition, vegetarians eat larger portions of foods that contain phytate. Phytate binds minerals such as zinc and strongly inhibits absorption. Vegetarians may require up to 50 percent more zinc than non-vegetarians to maintain adequate levels.

How Much and How Often

Zinc is an essential trace element. Our bodies do not store zinc for long, which is why you need a fresh supply at least every other day. Fortunately, you only need a little to achieve optimal cellular performance. The RDA for zinc is 11 mg for men, and 8 mg for women. The daily tolerable upper intake (UL) is 40 mg for men and women. I alternate between 15 mg and 25 mg four or five days per week. The 15 mg capsule also contains 1 mg of copper.

If you are mildly to moderately zinc-deficient and increase your daily intake, you may begin to notice results in just a few days. Results may include a stronger libido, leaner muscle tone, and better performance at the gym. Long-term results will include enhanced vitamin D utilization, faster healing of injuries, fewer illnesses, and healthier skin. Due to zinc's short shelf-life within our system, consider eating zinc-rich foods or taking low-dose supplements three to five days per week.

Do not mega-dose on zinc. Studies[48] have shown that excessive zinc intake can cause a variety of neurological and physiological problems, including high blood pressure. High blood pressure increases your risk of cardiac arrest and stroke. Continuous exposure to high levels of zinc can be extremely hazardous to your health.

A daily zinc intake of 40 mg or more can result in copper deficiency. Lower doses of zinc do not appear to diminish copper absorption. If you do not tolerate zinc well on an empty stomach, take it with a meal or try a different type.

High levels of zinc can also result in hair loss. Several zinc supplements are sold in 30 mg doses, which is a bit high if taken daily. Consider taking the full dose only three days per week (Monday, Wednesday, Friday), or breaking the tablet in half to take up to six days per week. The goal is to attain mineral balance.

Ingesting vitamins and minerals within an adequate range enables the body to better regulate the balance by metabolizing what it needs while excreting the rest. When you flood your system with one or two substances, it will have a more difficult time maintaining the necessary balance for maximum cellular potential. This is especially true when it comes to bone health.

Table 7. Zinc–Food

Food Type and Quantity	How Often
oysters, cooked (3 ounces).	Twice per week.
beef chuck roast, braised (3 ounces). crab, Alaska king, cooked (3 ounces). beef patty, broiled (3 ounces). breakfast cereal, fortified with 25 percent of the DV for zinc (¾ cup serving).	One serving of any of these food items, once or twice per day, four to seven days per week. Always consider calories and fat intake.

Table 8. Zinc–Supplement

Suggested Supplement Options	How Much and How Often
Jarrow Formulas–Zinc Balance: Zinc (15 mg) Copper (1 mg). Swanson–Zinc Orotate (10 mg). Liquid Ionic Zinc (various vendors) – (10 drops = 15 mg). Whole Foods 365 – Zinc (15 mg) Copper (1 mg). Solgar–Zinc Picolinate (22 mg).	4 to 6 days per week. Or a combination of foods (listed above) and supplements. 5 drops of ionic zinc 3 to 5 days per week can be considered for children.
Pure Encapsulations – Zinc 30: Zinc Picolinate (30 mg). Kal – Zinc Orotate (30 mg).	3 to 5 days per week. Excessive zinc depletes other minerals and may cause psychological problems.

Absorption Inhibitors

Phytate—present in foods such as cereals, corn, and rice—inhibits zinc absorption to some degree. Iron or calcium supplements, if taken together with zinc, can have an adverse effect on zinc absorption. No effect on zinc bioavailability appears to occur from naturally occurring iron, such as that found within red meat. Some medications, such as antibiotics and diuretics, can also inhibit zinc absorption.

Absorption Enhancers

Meat-based protein such as beef, turkey, chicken, eggs, and seafood enhance zinc absorption. These foods also help to counteract absorption inhibitors.

Best Formulation

- Zinc Orotate (absorbs exceptionally well; not easily impaired by phytate).
- Zinc monomethionine (absorbs extremely well; not easily impaired by phytate).
- Zinc picolinate (absorbs extremely well; may irritate empty stomach).
- Zinc citrate (absorbs well; may irritate empty stomach).
- Zinc gluconate (absorbs well; may irritate empty stomach).
- Zinc Balance consists of 15 mg of chelated zinc monomethionine and 1 mg of copper in a popular formulation called Opti-Zinc.
- Ionic (liquid) zinc.

Listen to Your Body

Symptoms of zinc deficiency can be easily misinterpreted or misdiagnosed. A compromised immune system resulting in frequent coughs or colds, sinus or respiratory infections, slow healing, or fatigue may be due to zinc deficiency. Mood swings, depression, ADHD, and difficulties with learning may also be symptoms of zinc deficiency. Zinc deficiency can also result in low testosterone or diminished thyroid function, which in turn can cause associated issues.

Very high levels of zinc can result in hair loss, nausea, vomiting, loss of appetite, diarrhea, abdominal cramps, and headaches. Mega-dosing on zinc will cause mineral imbalances, triggering mental and physical health problems. Additionally, excessive zinc can cause hypertension (high blood pressure).

Again, zinc supplementation taken with an evening meal or snack will enhance libido within an hour for the remainder of the night. This applies to men and women. However, as tempting as it may become, do not take excessive amounts of zinc.

Warning

High-dose zinc intake significantly inhibits copper absorption and mildly inhibits iron absorption. You may also wish to consider slightly increasing iron intake via food or periodic supplementation when increasing zinc intake. Iron supplementation can be extremely hazardous and should not be taken lightly. Consult with your physician.

Testing

- A zinc taste test may be an indicator of chronic zinc deficiency. Zinc sulfate is tasted, and your doctor will consider your response. It is convenient yet very subjective.
- A zinc serum test is more conventional. Unfortunately, several factors can cause inaccurate results.
- Blood plasma can offer an estimate of zinc levels in tissue. Cell levels are more useful as a measure of zinc nutritional status.
- Trial zinc supplementation at doses of 12–25 mg, four to five days per week, for a period of four to six weeks may reveal an existing zinc deficiency.

Vitamin D3

Impacts: Estrogen, Bone Health, Cancer, Diabetes, Osteoporosis, Depression, Weight Loss, Dementia, Alzheimer's, Blood Pressure, Multiple Sclerosis, Autoimmune Diseases, Mortality, Heart Health, Flu

Many individuals are aware of vitamin D's role in maintaining healthy bones and in the prevention of osteoporosis. What may come as news to some is the fact that calcitriol, the active derivative of vitamin D, is a critical hormone that is needed to support many biological functions, including the production of other hormones. It also provides protection against colon, prostate, and breast cancer. In addition, vitamin D is vital for maintaining a strong immune system.[49] 1,200 IU (International Units) of daily vitamin D3 supplementation has been shown to prevent respiratory infections and the flu.[50]

As mentioned in the previous discussion regarding magnesium, the vitamin D conversion process is amazing (see Figure 3 below). When you consume vitamin D (which is the first stage of the process), it is absorbed into your system (the second stage). It sits dormant inside your system and is eventually bound to a specific protein (third stage). That protein escorts vitamin D into your liver (fourth stage). Using magnesium and other cofactors, your liver converts the vitamin D you consumed (or developed via sun exposure) into 25-

hydroxyvitamin D [25(OH)D] (fifth stage). You are not done yet: this converted form of D is mostly inactive, meaning your body still has work to do.

Figure 3. Vitamin D Metabolic Process

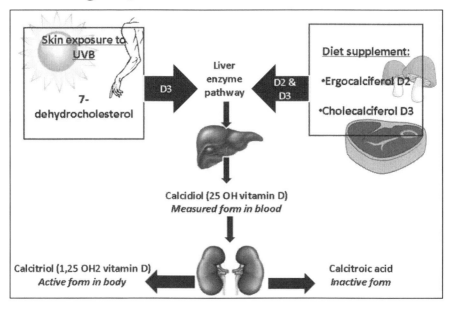

A diagram illustrating the different sources and forms of vitamin D. Retrieved February 17, 2019. *Journal of Advanced Research.*

The newly converted yet mostly dormant 25-hydroxyvitamin D [25(OH)D] is then circulated through your kidneys (sixth stage). Once there, it is converted yet again into 1,25-dihydroxyvitamin D [1,25(OH)2 D], also called calcitriol, its active hormonal form. Then, and only then, does the vitamin D you consume or develop from sun exposure perform its multitude of important tasks, such as increasing your calcium absorption rate, stimulating your production of osteoblasts, powering your immune system, and regulating the production of other hormones. Calcitriol also generates DNA sequencing for the creation of more osteocalcin, your bone-material binding element.[51,52] Calcitriol also increases testosterone levels.[53] In turn, testosterone improves bone density.

Vitamin D conversion is a complex procedure, and as such, is an extremely critical component of the overall bone-building process. Given this knowledge, we can hopefully better appreciate the need for high-value nutrients to fuel and feed the bone-building process. Interestingly, calcitriol can be bad for your bones under certain conditions. According to the Vitamin D Council:

> "Unlike 25(OH)D, calcitriol in the blood is an adaptive hormone; it is inversely related to the amount of calcium in the intestine. If there is no calcium in the intestine, calcitriol levels go up to remove calcium from bone, making osteoporosis worse. If calcium is present in sufficient quantities in the intestine, that calcium is absorbed and activated vitamin D levels fall."[54]

As I continually state, ingesting massive amounts of vitamin D3 is not the best strategy for maintaining adequate levels of the active hormone it eventually becomes. Excessive alcohol consumption diminishes liver function, which, in turn, can impede vitamin D conversion. Zinc and magnesium are cofactors in vitamin D absorption and conversion. Low levels of either can hinder the process.

Vitamin D deficiency has been linked to obesity[55] and several chronic illnesses. A large cohort study[56] associated vitamin D deficiency with all-cause mortality, cardiovascular diseases, cancer, and respiratory diseases. Vitamin D deficiency is also linked to a significantly greater risk of dementia and Alzheimer's disease.[57] Additionally, vitamin D can increase the rate at which the arteries harden if adequate vitamin K2 levels are not maintained. Nutrient balance is essential.

Once you correct a magnesium, zinc, and vitamin D deficiency, you can literally go without additional D3 intake for nearly two months without your cells knowing the difference.[58,59] Chance encounters between an individual's arms/face and direct sunlight produce 200 IU of vitamin D.[60] Certain ethnic groups, such as African Americans, require more prolonged exposure to obtain the same levels.

Two types of vitamin D supplementation are commonly used: ergocalciferol (D2) and cholecalciferol (D3).[61] Multiple studies concluded that vitamin D2 should no longer be used as a supplement or for fortification purposes.[62,63] Vitamin D3 is much more compatible with the human body's needs.

Although we have examined various forms of vitamin D related to the liver and kidney conversion process, there is one additional form: calcitroic acid. Calcitroic acid is produced from excess 25(OH)D, the substance produced by your liver, and excreted in the urine and bile.

Vegetarians

Vitamin D derived from plants is in the form of D2. D3 is derived from sun exposure and food sources, such as eggs, milk, and fish. Therefore, it may be necessary to supplement vitamin D3 more frequently, or at slightly higher dosages.

Myths and Misinformation

Charlotte, England – Sunday 12 March 2017:

"Unproven claims that vitamin D can cure a range of medical conditions are leading people to overdose with pills bought online, experts say. Hundreds of people in the UK are regularly taking toxic overdoses of vitamin D in supplements bought online, according to Britain's leading testing laboratory

Dr. Jonathan Berg, who runs the clinic, told *The Times*: 'We do a lot of vitamin D tests for the public, some of whom are taking huge amounts of vitamin D from the internet.'

'We're phoning people two or three times a week saying, "Your vitamin D is way higher than it should be. We suggest you come off whatever you're taking and see your GP." We've picked up hundreds of people who are overdosing themselves on vitamin D.'" [64]

As indicated in the preceding article, the internet has been flooded with short-sighted and misleading information regarding vitamin D. Some have taken an extreme view and suggest ingesting daily supplemental doses as high as 10,000 IU (300,000 IU a month). High-dose advocates either do not know or do not appreciate the complexities and nuances of your body's vitamin D hormone factory.

One very popular (commercial) doctor with a large internet platform implies it is necessary to obtain 8000 IU of vitamin D3 each day (240,000 IU a month). Coincidently, this individual also markets vitamin D3 and other supplements in his name. Various falsehoods and partial truths about vitamin D permeate the internet. We are going to address three of the most prevalent and extreme views.

> **Myth 1:** you need to consume more vitamin D to increase your measured vitamin D levels.

Extremely misleading. Vitamin D levels are not determined (medically) by the amount you ingest; they are measured by the amount of 25(OH)D that has been processed in the liver. Therefore, for many, there are more effective ways to increase this second form of vitamin D (as discussed in the "*Approach to Vitamin D Deficiency*" segment to follow). In many instances, consuming more vitamin D will not address the underlying cause of a vitamin D deficiency. The weak link is often in the absorption or conversion process; this can be due to lifestyle choices or a lack of something other than vitamin D, such as magnesium or zinc.

Exceptions to this include individuals with a genetic or medical condition; elderly individuals, or individuals who take certain medications, may also need higher amounts of supplementation. Condition-based risk factors for osteoporosis are contained in Chapter 2. Many of the risk factors listed involve some impairment to vitamin D utilization within the body.

Consuming more vitamin D on a short-term basis will correct a diagnosed vitamin D deficiency more quickly; however, this is not a long-term solution for otherwise healthy individuals. If the goal is to increase the level of 25(OH)D, this can be accomplished by resolving magnesium and zinc deficiencies and by improving liver function. These strategies will naturally result in higher 25(OH)D levels and address a multitude of other health issues without consuming massive amounts of vitamin D3. Again, this statement is not absolute as there will always be exceptions.

Myth 2: the average person should supplement 5,000 to 10,000 IU of D3 each day.

False. A 35-year-long osteoporosis study conducted in Canada demonstrated that **43.9 percent** of the participants who did not take vitamin D supplements during the spring and winter measured less than 50 nmol/L of 25(OH)D year-round. However, only **10 percent** of the participants who supplemented just **400 IU** (or more) of vitamin D a day measured less than 50 nmol/L of 25(OH)D year-round. The study focused on 577 men and 1,335 women. [65]

The myth of the need to ingest up to 10,000 IU of vitamin D supplements a day is primarily driven by an erroneous correlation between vitamin D3 developed internally from sun exposure, and vitamin D3 obtained through supplementation. This overly simplistic view ignores significant differences between the two processes.

It is true that under the right conditions (and if you do not bathe), twenty to thirty minutes of full skin exposure to direct sunlight can produce up to 10,000 IU of vitamin D3 in a healthy person. This is the first form of vitamin D, which is dormant. However, it takes up to two days after the skin's exposure to sunlight for that D3 to reach its highest concentration inside of your system. Then, it takes an additional three days for it to decrease below its serum "half-life" concentration, and even more time to completely dissipate. [66]

In basic terms, it takes nearly a week for vitamin D3 obtained through the skin to fully develop, and then pass through your system. Conversely, a vitamin D3 supplement will be absorbed into your system for processing within a few hours. If you could take a 10,000 IU slow-release supplement that took five days or more to absorb fully, you would be closer to duplicating the natural process. This alone should cause individuals to rethink this erroneous apples-to-oranges comparison.

There is another flaw associated with directly correlating D3 obtained from supplements with D3 acquired through sun exposure. Most of the vitamin D (precursor) created by sun exposure exists as oil on your skin. In fact, many D3 supplements are derived from the oil on sheep's wool. When you bathe (or shower), you wash off the remainder of the vitamin D-laden oil before your body absorbs it.

Myth 3: high levels of D3 supplementation is better for you.

Misleading. Under certain conditions, higher levels of vitamin D supplementation, such as 3000-10,000 IU a day, may be warranted. Individuals who suffer from an impaired conversion process—because of genetics, medications, age, or less than optimal liver or kidney function—may require higher daily intake.

However, gold-standard studies identify several harmful effects from consuming too much vitamin D, some of which can be deadly. Terms often used to describe the cause of these harmful side effects are Vitamin D Toxicity, and Hypervitaminosis D. Vitamin D Toxicity may occur from ingesting 10,000 to 40,000 IU/day.

Moreover, low levels and very high levels of 25(OH)D have been associated with an increased risk of various forms of cancer. [67] An intake of 5000 IU/day (without addressing other deficiencies) results in 40–60 ng/ml. I do not recommend exceeding 2000 IU of supplemental vitamin D a day (on average) after correcting a magnesium and zinc deficiency, which should also increase 25(OH)D levels. Consult with a licensed, medical professional before taking large quantities of vitamin D.

The other issue with excessive-D supplementation is the point of diminished returns. Studies have demonstrated 10,000 IUs of D3 supplementation results in nearly 100 ng/ml (with some variance) of serum level 25(OH)D, which is very high. **The studies, however, did not include increased magnesium and zinc intake, which significantly amplify your body's D3 utilization.** I suspect, had the study participants been given 400 mg of magnesium and 20 mg of zinc, their 25(OH)D serum levels would have gone much higher than 100 ng/ml. This is one of the biggest problems with viewing vitamin D (or any) supplementation in a vacuum. Nutrients are synergetic. They work in harmony to deliver a collective outcome. Adjusting the level of one nutrient can impact the level of another inside of your body.

Truth and Reality

As stated earlier, the vitamin D3 you consume is not measured to determine the levels in your blood serum. What is commonly measured is the converted form that is produced inside of the liver, 25(OH)D.[68] Why is this important?

Imagine your body as a car that usually gets thirty miles to the gallon. Obviously, this means that ten gallons of gasoline will provide three hundred miles of distance before you require a refill. One day, you notice that you are only getting one hundred miles of distance from ten gallons of gasoline. Would you just add more gas each day to make up the difference, or would you view this as an indicator that the engine may not be functioning correctly?

Now consider a scenario where your body normally produces 40 ng/ml of 25(OH)D whenever you obtain 1000 IU of vitamin D3. A few years later your body only produces 20 ng/ml of 25(OH)D, yet you are still obtaining 1000 IU of vitamin D3. Should you simply increase your vitamin D3 intake, or should you evaluate this issue more thoroughly to see if there is something going wrong in the conversion process? According to some, you should simply consume more vitamin D3 and move on. I disagree with that approach.

The bottom line is this: if you are supplementing an average of 1200-2000 IU of vitamin D3 per day and not maintaining a healthy level of the converted 25(OH)D in your system, this may indicate something is not working correctly inside your "engine." Of course, there are always exceptions. For instance, certain medications can interfere with your ability to metabolize vitamin D. Individuals aged seventy and older may also require a larger intake. An individual may undergo a change in work conditions (such as being reassigned to nightshift).

Consuming more D3 will likely improve your 25(OH)D levels, just as adding more gasoline to a compromised engine will allow you to drive farther. Unfortunately, it may also mask other issues that, if left untreated, can weaken your bones and damage your health.

In addition, high levels of calcitriol (1,25(OH)2D) (active D hormone) can raise serum calcium levels, which leads to vascular and tissue calcification and subsequent damage to the heart, blood vessels, and kidneys.[69] With relatively few exceptions, no healthy individual, regardless of the season or their location, requires more than 2000 IU of supplemental vitamin D a day from all sources, including multivitamins, standalone softgels, etc. (assuming they have corrected other vitamin deficiencies discussed earlier). With that said, as a military veteran, I support an individual's right to disagree with me.

Some only associate the term "healthy" with not catching the common cold or flu. This book's discussion is focused on the health of organs, bones, and internal processes. If a person is healthy internally, they should not require massive doses of supplemental D3 to maintain adequate levels of the active hormone. If they do need massive doses to sustain adequate hormone levels, then something inside of them is not working correctly. Our goal should always be to identify the weak link— be it a stressed or injured liver, compromised kidney function, a mineral cofactor deficiency, or something else—and hopefully correct the deficiency rather than mask it.

You may not realize that you have a "smart body," that readily adapts under normal circumstances. When your body detects enough active vitamin D in your system, it counteracts or shuts off its natural D production derived from sun exposure. This process is referred to as photochemical regulation.[70,71,72,73] Additionally, your body excretes less vitamin D in urine when your stores are low and more when your stores are high. If your body says it has had enough by down-cycling its vitamin D hormone production and flushing what it can down the toilet, should individuals saturate their system with massive doses of D3 based on information obtained from an internet blog?

How Much and How Often

Current RDA values for vitamin D are 600 IU for everyone except children younger than twelve months old (400 IU) and adults older than seventy-one (800 IU). These values represent the total intake throughout the day from multiple sources, not from a single food or supplement.

Evidence suggests the RDA for vitamin D may be enough to keep you alive and functional, but too low for optimal health.[74] 8,400-14,000 IU per week (an average of 1,200-2000 IU a day) is a safe target range for healthy adults who do not obtain enough sun exposure until further studies are conducted. If you go a little bit over or under, that should be perfectly fine. The closer you live to the equator, the less supplemental D3 you should need. Also, those of us near the halfway mark between the equator and the poles may require closer to 1600 IUs in the winter and little to no supplementation in the summer, assuming you love the sun! That said, taking 2000 IUs twice per week during the summer wouldn't hurt. Note that these are very general rules of thumb and do not cover all variables and conditions.

If you take a multivitamin, it will include vitamin D. Calcium products, such as Citracal, also contain vitamin D. Many of the foods you eat and the liquids you drink also provide vitamin D in conjunction with what is obtained through direct sun exposure.

Don't forget that maintaining optimal magnesium and zinc levels will exponentially increase vitamin D absorption, conversion, and utilization. When you add a common-sense approach to improving liver function—discussed later in Chapter 8—your vitamin D utilization will finally reach its full potential. This comprehensive, yet straightforward approach will be a significant step toward improving your system's bone-building productivity.

Approach to Vitamin D Deficiency

For decades, vitamin D deficiency has only been viewed as a problem to be resolved. In 1933, this was so because of a disease called rickets. Fortifying milk with vitamin D substantially reduced the incidence of the disease.

Unfortunately, the mindset of viewing vitamin D deficiency solely as a problem to be solved lingers, even today. We need to adjust contemporary thinking and view vitamin D deficiency as a potential symptom of a larger health issue. The challenge is overcoming the fact that consuming more vitamin D often does resolve the deficiency, resulting in a "problem solved" attitude—although the underlying health risk has not been identified yet.

To address common factors that may result in a medically diagnosed vitamin D deficiency, one might consider taking 100 to 200 mg of highly bioavailable magnesium two or three times per day in conjunction with 2,000 to 2,500 IU of D3 twice per day—or any dosage prescribed by a licensed physician—for a predetermined duration. I would encourage the caregiver to also add 15 to 30 mg of zinc for a comprehensive approach.[75] Regardless of the results, I would reduce zinc intake levels within a few weeks to 10–25 mg four or five days per week. Although the slightly higher dose is likely safe, too much zinc over extended periods can cause adverse neurological symptoms.

Additionally, to mitigate the risk of arterial calcification, 100 to 250 mcg of vitamin K2 (MK-7) should be included with treatment. This is mainly due to the restoration of D3 and magnesium levels, which will significantly enhance calcium absorption and utilization.

This comprehensive approach would not only resolve the vitamin D deficiency, but would also resolve and prevent a myriad of underlying health issues. Additionally, it will turbo-charge your bone-building engine. The information provided here should not be viewed as licensed medical advice. Rather, these are points to consider discussing with your physician if you have questions regarding vitamin D deficiency.

If you like, take this book with you and ask your doctor to read this chapter to aid in diagnosis. Most importantly, be willing to listen to that professional's counsel. Your doctor is far better equipped to advise you than I am (and is certainly better than some internet blog.) Your doctor knows you and your medical history; bloggers and I do not.

Table 9. Vitamin D3–Food

Food Type and Quantity	How Often
Cod liver oil, 1 tablespoon (1,360 IU).	One serving of any of these items once a day.
Swordfish, cooked, 3 ounces (566 IU).	
Salmon (sockeye), cooked, 3 ounces (447 IU).	Always consider calories and fat intake.

Table 10. Vitamin D3–Supplement

Suggested Supplement Options	How Much and How Often
Life Extension – D3 (1,000 IU).	One serving 3 to 5 days per week (you obtain D3 from multiple sources) or a combination of foods (listed above) and supplements.
Nutrigold – D3 (2,000 IU).	
Sports Research – D3 (2,000 IU).	

Absorption Inhibitors

Vitamin D production through exposure to sunlight is impeded by sunscreen. Conditions that affect digestion can reduce vitamin D absorption. Kidney disease and certain medications also inhibit the absorption of vitamin D. Glass acts as a barrier between your skin and sunlight, preventing vitamin D synthesis from occurring.

Absorption Enhancers

Vitamin D is a fat-soluble nutrient. Taking vitamin D3 with a meal increases absorption significantly. Vitamin D3 is more effective at raising serum levels when not taken every day. Smaller doses (2,000 IU or less) are absorbed more fully than large doses. Magnesium activates vitamin D after it has been absorbed. Zinc is also a cofactor for vitamin D absorption.

Best Formulation

- Vitamin D3 (highly compatible with the human body).

Nutrigold D3 is natural, sourced from lanolin, encapsulated in organic olive oil, and is GMO-free. It is available in doses of 1,000, 2,000, and 5,000 IU. Other reputable manufacturers are also worth considering.

Personal

My weekly supplemental intake of vitamin D typically falls between 10,000–14,000 IU. I consume one D3 softgel (1000 IU) four days per week in conjunction with one or two Citracal-Petites (250-500 IU) five or six days per week. I also take a multivitamin (1000 IU) and enjoy organic milk, meals, and sunshine. I assume a 65-75 percent supplement absorption rate.

Listen to Your Body

Vitamin D deficiency may compromise the immune system, resulting in symptoms such as frequent coughs and colds, sinus or respiratory infections, slow healing, and fatigue. Vitamin D deficiency may also present itself as poor density and structure in bones and teeth.

Symptoms of Vitamin D toxicity do not manifest until several months after excessive doses of vitamin D are consumed. Symptoms and side effects of vitamin D toxicity include: fatigue, nausea, vomiting, polyuria, polydipsia, weakness, constipation, confusion, abnormal heart rhythm, nervousness, pruritus, proteinuria, urinary casts, azotemia, metastatic calcifications in soft tissue, and renal failure.

Warning

Taking vitamin D supplements without adequate vitamin K2 may increase the risk of developing cardiovascular disease. The most common adverse effects of vitamin D supplementation are hypercalcemia and hypercalciuria. African Americans, nightshift workers, and seniors should have their vitamin D levels tested more frequently than other individuals.

High serum levels of vitamin D are associated with a greater risk of cancer, cardiovascular events, and more falls and fractures among the elderly.

Testing

The Vitamin D Council[76] (VDC) lists three ways to get tested:

1. Ask your doctor for a vitamin D test. Be specific and ask for a 25(OH)D test. The 25(OH)D test is the only one that will tell you whether you're getting enough vitamin D.

2. In-home tests are sent to your residence. You prick your finger and put a drop of blood on blotter paper. You then send the paper to a laboratory to be tested. Companies that offer in-home tests include:
   - ZRT Labs. The Vitamin D Council works with ZRT Labs.
   - New Century Diagnostics via Home Health Testing.
   - City Assays. They are based in the UK and offers the cheapest test internationally. It takes about ten days for the test to arrive in the USA.

3. Order a test online. A lab will process your blood work.

CHAPTER EIGHT

Liver & Kidney Health

Rarely discussed is the hugely significant role the liver plays in bone quality and density. Kidneys are key players as well, but often do not take the same level of abuse as the liver. A healthy liver is the heart and soul of bone health. Individuals suffering from liver disease are keenly aware of this. Many liver diseases, such as nonalcoholic fatty liver disease (NAFLD), display no noticeable symptoms and go undiagnosed. The same is true of kidney diseases.

You have just learned that the vitamin D you eat, drink, or obtain from the sun is dormant and does nothing for you until it is converted. You also learned that this dormant form of vitamin D enters the liver to be converted into 25-hydroxyvitamin D [25(OH)D]. Although this converted form is still mostly inactive, this crucial step allows the final conversion of vitamin D into the active hormone your bones so desperately need.

Diminished liver or kidney function adversely impacts vitamin D conversion and the production of other important hormones, such as osteoprotegerin (OPG).[77] In turn, reduced levels of these critical substances drastically impede the production of healthy bone material. Taking care of your liver is extremely beneficial for building strong bones and maintaining multiple facets of your health.

Alcohol abuse can cause cirrhosis of the liver, thereby diminishing your bone-building capacity to a great extent. Constant intake of processed food and poorly prepared fatty meals can result in a fatty liver, diminishing your bone-building capacity. Again, no individual will ever achieve a perfect diet. The goal here is to be mindful of how important your liver is to your bone quality, life expectancy, and overall health. If you drink alcoholic beverages, do so in moderation.

A ten-year study published in Hepatology (2014) shows liver injury caused by herbals and dietary supplements (HDS) has increased from 7 percent to 20 percent. Green tea extract (camellia sinensis) has been identified as a significant cause of liver injury. Many retailers boast of having high concentrations of this ingredient in their products to burn fat.

A searchable database for harmful products is located at the following website for the NIH. Visit the following links for additional details. URL addresses may change over time.

- https://livertox.nlm.nih.gov/Hydroxycut.htm
- https://livertox.nlm.nih.gov

Many of your body's nutrients are stored in the liver; such as vitamin A, D, E, and K. Overwhelming your liver with excessive amounts of any substance will not make it perform better. Everything in the human body has a breakover threshold, meaning adding more of substance X will yield diminishing returns and can eventually be harmful.

Drug-Induced Liver Injury Network (DILIN)

The National Institute of Diabetes and Digestive and Kidney Diseases (NIDDK) established the DILIN to evaluate the impact of medications and dietary supplements on the liver. The main results of their 10-year study is cited below.

> "Liver injury due to herbal and dietary supplements (HDS) increased from 7% to 20% during the study period. Bodybuilding HDS caused prolonged jaundice (median 91 days) in young men but did not result in any fatalities or liver transplantation. The remaining HDS cases presented as hepatocellular injury, predominantly in middle-aged women and more frequently led to death or transplantation compared to injury from medications."[78]

More information about the DILIN is available at:

- https://dilin.org/

Center for Drug Evaluation and Research (CDER)

According to its website, the Food and Drug Administration's (FDA) Center for Drug Evaluation and Research (CDER) promotes and protects the health of Americans by ensuring that all prescription and over-the-counter drugs are safe and effective. CDER evaluates all new drugs before they are sold and serves as a consumer watchdog for the more than ten thousand drugs on the market to ensure they continue to meet the highest standards.

The Center routinely monitors TV, radio, and print drug ads to ensure they are truthful and balanced. CDER also plays a critical role in providing health professionals and consumers with information, enabling them to use drugs appropriately and safely.

Please visit CDER for a current list of tainted supplements at:

- https://tinyurl.com/mg232tg

According to CDER, the list of 923 tainted products in their database as of February 7, 2019 reflect only a small fraction of the potentially hazardous products marketed to consumers. Even if a product is not included in this list, consumers should exercise caution before using certain products.

Pamper Your Liver

One of the best and simplest approaches to protect your liver (besides ending bad habits) is to drink a glass of lemon water from time to time—perhaps once per week. Some suggest doing so more frequently.

Simply cut a fresh lemon, add a few slices into a glass of room-temperature water (squeeze the juice into the water first), and allow it to sit for several minutes, then enjoy! Please note that the acidic nature of lemons can erode tooth enamel over time. It is recommended that you use a straw, rinse after drinking, or brush your teeth when you are done.

Other than lemon water, there are several foods and beverages available to you that can pamper your liver. The list includes green tea (not extract), grapefruit (and juice), beets (and juice), broccoli, Brussels sprouts, mustard greens, walnuts, fatty fish (not fried), blueberries, and cranberries (including juice). Add a few (or all) of these food and beverage items to your menu as often as you like. A byproduct of eating healthier is reduced levels of toxins in your system, which is great.

Also, organic produce has been shown to decrease the level of chemical toxins in individuals. However, organic food is often far more expensive than other produce, meaning some people simply cannot afford it. Nevertheless, you are encouraged to add some or all of the products previously listed to your diet, even if you opt for non-organic varieties.

Bone health is not an all-or-nothing process. Any improvements you can reasonably accomplish for your liver will help your bone quality and overall health. Simply do what you can.

CHAPTER NINE

Calcium

Impacts: Bone Health, Heart Health, Nervous System, Blood Clotting, Cancer

Calcium supports a wide variety of cellular activities. Almost all calcium is stored in bones and teeth, where it supports their structure and hardness. The body needs calcium for muscle movement, normal heart function, and to allow nerves to transmit messages between the brain and the rest of the body. Calcium deficiency has also been linked to forms of cancer.[79]

Calcium deficiency can cause you to feel fatigued and less energetic. You may also encounter muscle tremors (spasms) with or without muscle cramps. Low calcium levels can cause numbness or tingling (pins and needles) sensations. Moreover, calcium deficiency can interfere with sleep and cause you to gain weight.

High-dosage, long-term calcium supplementation can be detrimental to your health. Studies indicate excessive calcium intake increases incidents of heart disease and (possibly) cancer while doing little to improve bone health.

Every individual requires adequate calcium intake for optimum health. The trick is to obtain the correct amount of calcium you need and to process that calcium in a beneficial (not detrimental) way. An archived article on WebMD[80] cites Gary G. Schwartz, PhD with the following statement:

> "Many of your body's functions run on calcium, just like your laptop runs on electricity," Schwartz says. "Too little calcium in the blood can cause convulsions and too much can lead to a coma. Since your body cannot afford to oscillate between convulsions and coma, the range of serum calcium is tightly controlled."

Before your body can fully utilize calcium, you need the proper levels of vitamin D to absorb it. Before vitamin D can effectively help you absorb calcium, you need a healthy liver and healthy kidneys. Adequate levels of magnesium and zinc are also required to maximize vitamin D performance.

Once calcium is absorbed, it requires a guide to direct it to your bones and teeth. Without that guide, calcium builds up inside your arteries over time, making blood circulation more difficult—even to the point of cardiac arrest or stroke. Vitamin K2 is that guide (see Chapter 5 on vitamin K2).

Bones also require phosphorus to complete their structure. However, too much phosphorus will force your bones to release calcium into your bloodstream, causing your bones to weaken over time. These and other components need to be in balance to optimize your bone structure and overall health.

Many people are not aware that we live in a phosphorus-heavy dietary environment; processed food in particular is high in phosphorus. Therefore, it may be prudent to engage in low-dose calcium supplementation and to add calcium-rich foods to your diet.

Keep in mind that you have likely improved calcium absorption and utilization by applying the information in this book. This alone should offset some or all of the negative effects to your bone health that may be caused by a high-phosphorus diet.

Calcium levels in our bodies will often decline as we age. As women age, their ability to absorb calcium may decrease due to reduced estrogen levels. Deficiencies in nutrients such as vitamin D, iodine, and zinc affect estrogen production. Therefore, maintaining proper levels of these critical elements serves to optimize bone health in more ways than one.

How Much and How Often

Calcium supplements come in various forms. Calcium carbonate requires stomach acid to be absorbed and must be taken with a meal. Calcium citrate, which can be more expensive, is more readily absorbed (with or without food). Many individuals may benefit from supplementing 200-500 mg of calcium four-to-seven times a week.

Concerns have been raised over the levels of heavy metals, such as lead and mercury, contained in coral calcium. A study on calcium supplements found concentrations of lead at 0.106-0.384 mg/kg in oysters, coral, and animal bone, which are considered sources of natural raw calcium. Traces of mercury and cadmium were also detected.

If you choose to supplement with coral calcium or a similar product, purchase it from a reputable manufacturer. Also, ensure the product has been tested for heavy metals and other hazardous elements, preferably by a trustworthy third party. The RDA for elemental calcium varies with age:

- Males and females ages nineteen to fifty (1,000 mg).
- Males ages fifty-one to seventy (1,000 mg).
- Females ages fifty-one to seventy (1,200 mg).
- Males and females age seventy-one and older (1,200 mg).

Please remember that this reflects your total calcium intake from food, drinks, and supplements. Never supplement 100 percent of the RDA for calcium unless directed to do so by your physician. Furthermore, you should not take calcium supplements without also maintaining adequate (not excessive) levels of K2.

Additionally, the information discussed in the previous chapters significantly enhances (or amplifies) your body's ability to absorb and utilize calcium. This alone increases your calcium intake. Therefore, if you apply what we have discussed thus far, you do not need to ingest excessive amounts of supplemental calcium.

Table 11. Calcium−Food

Food Type and Quantity	How Often
Kale.	One serving of any of these items twice a day.
Broccoli.	
Milk.	
Yogurt.	Always consider calories and fat intake.
Cheese.	
Canned fish with soft bones (e.g., sardines, salmon).	
Orange juice (calcium fortified).	

Table 12. Calcium−Supplement

Suggested Supplement Options	How Much and How Often
Citracal Petites – Calcium Citrate (200 mg) D3 (250 IU) each.	1 to 2 pills per day, 3 to 7 days per week.
Pure Encapsulations – Calcium Citrate (150 mg) each.	If 2 pills per day, consider taking separately.
BlueBonnet – Calcium Citrate (250 mg) D3 (200 IU) Magnesium Aspartate (100 mg) each.	Consult with your physician.
NATURELO – Plant-Based Calcium (150 mg) D3 (6.25 mcg) Magnesium Glycine (50 mg) each.	

Absorption Inhibitors

Caffeine; vitamin D deficiency; magnesium deficiency; foods with phytate, such as wheat bran, pinto beans, navy beans and peas; and foods that contain oxalates, such as beets, spinach, rhubarb, okra, tea, and sweet potatoes, inhibit calcium absorption.

Excessive protein and phosphorus consumption leaches calcium from your bones and may necessitate higher calcium intake (see following chapters on Phosphorus and Protein). Improper thyroid function can impede calcium absorption and utilization.

Absorption Enhancers

Vitamin D, vitamin K2, magnesium, and lysine greatly enhance the absorption and utilization of calcium. Note: when magnesium is included in a calcium supplement, calcium will inhibit magnesium absorption to some degree.

Best Formulation

- Calcium citrate (absorbs exceptionally well with food or on an empty stomach)
- Calcium carbonate (absorbs with food; less expensive than calcium citrate).

It may be prudent to only take one 200 mg pill once or twice per day rather than two simultaneously. Doing so will enable greater calcium absorption. However, it is always easier to take things together for fear of forgetting to take another later in the day. Do what works best with your lifestyle.

Citracal also makes a chewable calcium supplement. Other reputable manufacturers sell high-quality calcium supplements, such as Pure Encapsulations and Bluebonnet. Choose the one that is right for you. Don't forget your K2.

Personal Note

Citracal Petites previously recommended 800 mg (two pills twice per day). They currently recommend 400 mg (two pills once per day). I take one pill once or twice a day (200-400 mg) and consume calcium-rich foods such as organic milk, broccoli, and kale. I take vitamin K2 in the form of MK-7 to protect my arteries and maximize calcium utilization in my bones and teeth.

Listen to Your Body

Calcium deficiency can present itself as fatigue, muscle cramps, muscle tremors, muscle twitches, numbness, tingling (pins and needles) sensations, impaired sleep, or having difficulty losing weight. Excess calcium may result in symptoms such as constipation or kidney stones.

Warning

As stated earlier, do not exceed 600 mg of (elemental) calcium supplementation a day unless directed to do so by a physician. A lower dose is safer in the long run.

If a physician recommends supplementing more than 500 mg of calcium a day, discuss any concerns you may have regarding an increased risk of heart disease. In addition, ask your physician to consider looking at your magnesium levels, vitamin K2 intake, and vitamin D levels. As a reminder, magnesium testing using epithelial cell analysis appears to be far more accurate than testing via blood analysis. Be mindful of foods and products that inadvertently trigger the release of calcium from your bones into your bloodstream, such as excessive phosphorus or excessive protein.

Some discussion has been generated correlating excessive calcium levels with forms of cancer, especially prostate cancer. One major ten-year study found no correlation between high levels of calcium caused by supplements and cancer. This suggests a possible correlation between calcium derived from certain produce and elevated cancer risk. However, there is a mixed bag of results from multiple studies.

Don't panic. Don't go on a mad hunt for online articles. You must consider the totality of information versus the online views of a few individuals or organizations. For now, simply do all things in moderation and you should be fine. You need calcium. You do not need excessive amounts of calcium.

Testing

Blood serum tests for calcium levels are very common. A sublingual epithelial cell analysis[81] may be considered for measuring calcium levels within your tissue. The test kit is shipped to your local physician, who collects small soft tissue samples from the mouth. Individuals who have undergone the process state that the procedure is noninvasive and virtually painless. You are encouraged to engage in additional research before subjecting yourself to any testing procedure.

As mentioned previously, another calcium testing method worth strong consideration is the coronary calcium scan.[82] The coronary calcium scan looks for specks of calcium in the walls of the coronary (heart) arteries. There are two forms of the scan performed by two different machines—electron beam computed tomography (EBCT) and multidetector computed tomography (MDCT). Calcifications in the coronary arteries are an early sign of coronary heart disease (CHD).[83]

Checkpoint

(resolving D3 deficiency) + (healthy liver and kidneys) + (resolving calcium deficiency)

- leads to -

stronger and denser bone-building capability + improved immune response, estrogen levels, healing, heart function, weight control, mood, and more...

End Checkpoint

CHAPTER TEN

Phosphorus

Impacts: Bone Health, Blood Pressure, Heart Health, Weight Loss, Depression, Muscle Cramps, Menstrual Cramps, Diabetes, Protein Synthesis, Fatigue, Nervous System

Phosphorus is one of the most abundant substances inside your bones. It plays a critical role in supporting and maintaining numerous biological functions and is used to produce DNA and RNA inside of your cells. Phosphorus impacts brain function, muscle tissue, and organs. Proper phosphorus levels improve muscle endurance and help metabolize fat. It also promotes deeper and more restful sleep.

The human body is very proactive in preventing a phosphorus deficiency. It does so by reducing the amount of phosphorus that is excreted through your urine and reabsorbing it back into your system. This is one of the many amazing things that are constantly occurring inside of you.

According to a national survey,[84] the average woman ingests more than 1100 mg of phosphorus per day. The average man consumes over 1600 mg. As with sodium, phosphorous is a common food additive. The higher your processed food intake, the higher your daily phosphorus intake (due to phosphate additives).

High phosphorus consumption triggers a process that causes your bones to release calcium into your bloodstream. This interaction can weaken your bones. Also, high levels of phosphorus can combine with calcium and harden the interior lining of your arteries. This is especially true for those who do not have adequate levels of K2.

Individuals should try to reduce processed food consumption; however, this is often easier said than done. The good news is that if you maintain adequate levels of magnesium, vitamin D3, vitamin K2, and calcium, you can offset the potential harm resulting from the typical high-phosphorus diet.

How Much and How Often

The recommended daily allowances (RDA) for phosphorus are as follows:

Table 13 . Phosphorus RDA

Ages	Males (mg/day)	Females (mg/day)
1–3	460	460
4–8	500	500
9–13	1,250	1,250
14–18	1,250	1,250
19+	700	700

Phosphorus intake is typically too high in the average diet. Therefore, I do not recommend any form of supplementation beyond what may be contained in the average multivitamin.

If anything, you may wish to find ways to reduce your intake. However, do not become overly concerned. Every vitamin and mineral discussed thus far can significantly increase your body's calcium utilization, thereby reducing the impact of excess phosphorous to some degree.

Because of human factors, I suggest reasonable measures that can yield exponential, long-term results. Remember: anything you do in an informed, balanced way is an improvement. Do as much as you can for as long as you can. Also, be sure to reward yourself every so often and just live. After all, you should enjoy life, not fear it.

Table 14. Phosphorus–Food

Foods Containing Phosphorus (for informational purposes only)	
Salmon	Squash Seeds
Yogurt	Sunflower Seeds
Pumpkin Seeds	Almonds
Chicken	Sesame Seeds
Turkey	Soybeans
Beef	Flax Seeds

Supplementation

Phosphorus supplementation is not recommended without medical supervision.

Listen to Your Body

Symptoms of phosphorus deficiency include fatigue, anxiety, bone disorders, and hormone imbalances.

Warning

Do not ingest excessive amounts of phosphorus.

Testing

Blood serum tests for phosphate levels are the most common. One should also consider the sublingual epithelial cell analysis (EXA test). You are encouraged to perform additional research and consult with your physician before subjecting yourself to any procedure.

Iodine

Impacts: Metabolism, Fatigue, Depression, Immune System, Cancer, Bone Health, Fibrosis, Testosterone, Cholesterol, Coronary Artery Disease, Autoimmune Diseases, Hair Loss

Iodine is essential for proper thyroid function. Maintaining optimum thyroid function is critical to many aspects of your physical and mental well-being, including bone health. This ripple effect is how we come to appreciate iodine's role in combating osteoporosis and other ailments.

There are two overarching forms of improper thyroid function: hypothyroidism (a thyroid that does not produce enough thyroid hormone) and hyperthyroidism (a thyroid that produces excessive thyroid hormone). Excessive iodine intake has been directly linked to hyperthyroidism. Hyperthyroidism has been directly linked to low bone density as it causes your body to expel more of your body's phosphorous and calcium stores.

Beyond building stronger bones, iodine is a natural cancer fighting agent. Not only does it shrink cancer cells, it also causes apoptosis (automatic cell death) of some forms of cancer cells.

Myths and Misinformation

Even though the RDA for iodine is only 150 mcg (micrograms), some individuals ignited an iodine mega-dosing frenzy, suggesting supplementation of up to 12.5 mg (milligrams) per day. They suggest slowly increasing the dose to build a tolerance to their massive recommended amounts. It is possible the frenzy is tied to a miscalculation within a 1967 research paper that focused on iodine consumption in Japan.

Truth and Reality

Virtually all credible data strongly cautions against consuming large amounts of iodine. The potential for exposure to a radiological hazard, such as the aftermath of a nuclear explosion, is the exception. Excessive iodine intake will cause your thyroid to decrease its iodine absorption and your kidneys to eliminate more iodine via urine.

Individuals who are susceptible to thyroid dysfunction have triggered iodine-induced health issues, such as hypothyroidism. A detailed discussion of this topic and the report that has been used to fuel this misunderstanding is included in Chapter 18, "Supplement Abuse."

Vegetarians

Vegetarians and vegans are at greater risk of developing iodine deficiency than others. Soy and cruciferous vegetables such as cabbage, broccoli, cauliflower, and Brussels sprouts interfere with the utilization of iodine.[85]

How Much and How Often

The RDA for iodine in adults is 150 mcg. The upper limit is approximately 1 mg (1,000 mcg). In the rare event of a radiological incident (such as a nuclear explosion), the CDC recommends a single dose of 130 mg of potassium iodide for adults under forty years of age.

A 2009 study in Switzerland indicates that roughly half of the European population is mildly iodine deficient. A 2008 United States Food and Drug Administration (FDA) total diet study demonstrated that iodine intake levels in the United States ranged from 138 to 353 mcg per day.

Attaining proper iodine levels can yield both short- and long-term benefits. People who are extremely deficient may see results within a few weeks, including increased energy and weight loss. If you are not deficient, you may not feel any results. Positive results may occur very gradually over several months for mild iodine deficiencies. Skipping a day or two of supplementation enhances the absorption rate. Sounds odd, but it's true.

China's National Iodine Deficiency Disorders Elimination Program[86] decreased goiter rates among children from 20.4 percent to 8.8 percent in four years via iodized salt. The International Council for the Control of Iodine Deficiency Disorders (ICCIDD) Global Network[87] and the American Thyroid Association[88] confirm that 150 mcg of iodine is adequate for most adults (except during pregnancy).

Table 15. Iodine–Food

Food Type and Quantity	How Often
Sea vegetables. Cod. Turkey breast. Eggs. Milk. Yogurt. Cranberries. Navy beans. Potatoes (baked).	One serving of any of these items two or three times a day. Always consider calories and fat intake.

Table 16. Iodine–Supplement

Suggested Supplement Options	How Much and How Often
LL – Magnetic Clay Nascent Iodine - 1 oz. (400 mcg per drop). Go Nutrients – Iodine Edge Nascent Iodine (~300 mcg per drop). NOW – Kelp Caps (150 mcg).	1 drop, 1–2 days per week. 1 pill, 3–4 days per week. (Or a combination of foods and supplements.)

Absorption Inhibitors

Fluoride, chlorine, bromide (bromine, bromate), all of which are found in white flour, bread, rolls, soda, and tap water, inhibit the thyroid's ability to absorb iodine. Soy and cruciferous vegetables such as cabbage, broccoli, cauliflower, and Brussels sprouts also interfere with iodine absorption. Caffeine products may also inhibit iodine absorption.

Absorption Enhancers

Nascent (atomic) iodine absorbs exceptionally well on an empty stomach. Typically, the consumer must add a drop of liquid iodine to a glass of water and swallow. Nascent iodine can also be absorbed sublingually. It has been reported to be less toxic and better tolerated than other forms. There is no risk of heavy metals.

Molecular iodine supplements have grown in popularity and appear to absorb well on an empty stomach and moderately well with food. Be advised that some forms of molecular iodine are sold in extremely high doses.

Potassium iodide is primarily absorbed within the GI tract and is considered less effective than nascent iodine. Unless you have a properly diagnosed medical condition, a regimen of 75 to 150 mcg taken three-to-five days per week should serve to maintain your thyroid health. Remember, you are also obtaining iodine from other sources. This is a supplement, not a replacement.

Best Formulation

- Nascent (atomic) iodine (absorbs exceptionally well; superior form of iodine).
- Molecular iodine (absorbs well on an empty stomach).
- Potassium iodide (absorbs moderately well).
- Iodized salt is beneficial for maintaining proper iodine levels. Unfortunately, too much salt may lead to other health issues, such as hypertension.
- LL's Magnetic Clay Nascent Iodine (atomic iodine) is extremely effective.

Listen to Your Body

Iodine deficiency can cause impaired mental function, fatigue, goiter, or hypothyroidism (underactive thyroid). With hypothyroidism, you may feel colder and suffer memory lapses or even depression. Detailed symptoms are listed under "Hashimoto's Disease" on the following page.

Severe iodine deficiency during pregnancy can result in children with mental and growth disorders. Excessive iodine can cause hypothyroidism or hyperthyroidism (overactive thyroid), resulting in nervousness, irritability, anxiety, difficulty sleeping, perspiration, rapid heartbeat, hand tremors, brittle hair, and muscle fatigue.

Warning

On June 5, 2013, the American Thyroid Association[89] released a statement advising against the daily ingestion of iodine supplements in excess of 500 mcg. They further stated that consuming more than 1,100 mcg of iodine per day may cause thyroid dysfunction.

Long-term exposure to excessive levels of iodine can cause autoimmune diseases and thyroid cancer. Additionally, some iodine supplements derived from kelp may contain heavy metals. Supplement iodine with extreme caution. The thyroid gland influences every aspect of your health.

Testing

Urine analysis for iodine excretion levels is very common. A blood serum analysis, however, may yield more accurate results.

Due to the characteristics of iodine and various environmental factors, I remain skeptical about the validity of iodine skin tests as an indicator of an iodine deficiency. Additional testing methods are available.

Hashimoto's Disease

As stated by the Office on Women's Health,[90] Hashimoto's disease (Hashimoto's thyroiditis) is an autoimmune disease that affects the thyroid. Thyroid hormone levels are controlled by the pituitary gland inside the brain. It makes thyroid-stimulating hormone (TSH), which triggers the production of thyroid hormone. In those suffering from Hashimoto's disease, the immune system makes antibodies that damage thyroid cells and interfere with their ability to make thyroid hormone. **Excessive iodine can trigger Hashimoto's thyroiditis**

in people who are prone to getting it and occurs nearly seven times more frequently in women than men.

Over time, thyroid damage can cause thyroid hormone levels to be too low (hypothyroidism). An underactive thyroid causes every function of the body to slow down, including heart rate, brain function, and metabolism. Hashimoto's disease is the most common cause of an underactive thyroid. It is closely related to Graves' disease, another autoimmune disease that affects the thyroid.

Many people with Hashimoto's disease have no symptoms for years. An enlarged thyroid, called a goiter, is often the first sign of illness.

Symptoms of an underactive thyroid include:

- Fatigue
- Weight gain
- Pale, puffy face
- Feeling cold
- Joint and muscle pain
- Constipation
- Dry, thinning hair
- Heavy menstrual flow or irregular periods
- Depression
- A slowed heartrate
- Problems getting pregnant

CHAPTER TWELVE

Potassium

Impacts: Stress, Heart Health, Bone Health, Cancer, Insulin Resistance, Menopause, Insomnia, Infant Colic, Allergies, Headaches, Weight Loss Acne, Alzheimer's, Arthritis, Vision, Bloating, Fever, Gout, Irritability, Muscle Weakness, Muscular Dystrophy, Chronic Fatigue, Dermatitis

Potassium works as an electrolyte and is vital to every process that keeps us alive. It is also a direct contributor to the bone-building process.[91] Individuals with physically demanding lifestyles require more potassium than those without as they need to regularly replenish their supplies. Regularly obtaining the recommended daily adequate intake of 4,700 mg is next to impossible for most people. My hope is to get you close to the halfway mark of 2,350 mg, or even a little bit further. In the end, most individuals should do the best they can to increase their potassium intake, even if only by a few hundred additional milligrams each day.

Regardless of how beneficial obtaining 4,700 mg of potassium a day may be, few people would be able to do so for any length of time. The good news is that when you establish adequate levels of magnesium, the magnesium will improve your body's utilization of potassium. It does not make up the full difference between what you consume and the recommended 4,700 mg, but it does help.

Potassium intake is directly associated with bone mineral density (BMD). Research demonstrated that individuals with higher potassium intake maintained greater BMD, thus reducing their risk of developing osteoporosis.[92] Furthermore, increasing the potassium-sodium ratio within the human body resulted in fewer hip fractures.

Potassium participates in a multitude of life-giving functions, such as nerve impulse conduction, normal heart rhythm, and the regulation of blood glucose levels. It is also required to build muscle matter and to burn carbohydrates for energy. Potassium is essential for every muscle contraction in your body, including cardiac, skeletal, and smooth muscle tissue.

Potassium actively lowers blood pressure in people who suffer from hypertension. Hypertension dramatically increases your risk factor for cardiac arrest and stroke.

Health issues associated with sodium often result from an extremely low intake of potassium. Potassium helps you expel sodium via your urine. Of the various supplemental forms, potassium citrate is alkaline, potassium gluconate is pH neutral, and potassium chloride is acidic. Kidneys regulate potassium levels by excreting it through the urine. Drinking excess water depletes your potassium via urination.

Potassium citrate prevents and reduces kidney stones by adhering to calcium in the urine. Potassium citrate also prevents urine from becoming too acidic.

How Much and How Often

As previously stated, the daily adequate intake (AI) recommendation is 4,700 mg for adults, which roughly equates to eating twelve bananas per day. Low-sodium V8, pomegranate juice, and pure coconut water are excellent sources of potassium.

Supplemental potassium can be found in tablet, capsule, salt, and powder forms. Potassium pills are regulated not to exceed 99 mg of elemental potassium. High concentrations (in pill form) can irritate and/or damage portions of the stomach lining by remaining in direct contact with one area for extended periods. Potassium powder and salt, when added to food or liquid, is safer for your stomach lining at higher doses than pills. However, an extremely high dose of supplemental potassium can be harmful. I recommend not ingesting more than eight hundred milligrams of potassium salt at one time, unless directed to do so by a physician.

According to a five-year NHANES study comprised of 10,563 participants, the usual intake of sodium and potassium for American adults amounted to 3,569 mg/day (sodium) and 2,745 mg/day (potassium), reflecting a dietary ratio of 1.41:1. Based on this study, many adults need to consume an additional 1,880 mg of potassium a day to meet the recommended adequate intake (AI) level. This number is even higher for individuals who drink large amounts of water or engage in various forms of exercise. **Do not supplement more than 2,400 mg of potassium in a single day without consulting with a physician.** Consider adding potassium powder or salt to your meals and smoothies throughout the day. Again, consult with your physician as high levels of potassium in concentrated forms can cause stomach ulcers and other problems. This is especially true for individuals with compromised kidney function.

Supplemental potassium should always be taken with a meal to protect the stomach lining and induce a slower, more even absorption rate. If you weigh 160 pounds or more, I encourage you not to exceed 800 mg (powder or salt) in a single dose. I encourage individuals weighing less than 160 pounds not to exceed 5 mg (powder or salt) for each pound of body weight in a single dose. For example, an individual who weighs 125 pounds would not exceed 625 mg (5 mg X 125) in a single dose, unless directed to do so by a physician. Again, you are encouraged not to exceed 2400 mg of supplemental potassium in a single day, which can be accomplished in three or more separate doses with meals.

Admittedly, this approach may be overly cautious. When it comes to your health, a bit of caution is always warranted. Individuals with underlying health conditions such as impaired kidney function or compromised heart health should always consult with a physician before taking potassium supplements.

It is possible to unknowingly suffer from impaired kidney function, or some other undiagnosed condition, which may cause an otherwise safe dose of potassium to rise to dangerous levels.

Supplemental potassium can be absorbed more rapidly and more completely than food-based elements. For instance, 800 mg of potassium contained in two bananas is not absorbed in the same manner as 800 mg of supplemental potassium in a cup of water.

If you are potassium-deficient, you may notice results within two days to two weeks of increased intake, including fewer muscle cramps, a more relaxed respiratory system, and more endurance during physical activities. Long-term results could include denser bones, improved weight management, lower blood pressure, and improved heart function.

A combination of potassium-rich foods and beverages coupled with supplementation can help individuals improve their potassium levels. An informative article published in *Medical News Today* lists potassium-rich foods and their content.[93] I've added a few additional items to the list.

- Cooked, boiled, or drained beet greens, without salt – 1,309 mg.
- Canned white beans – 1,189 mg.
- Cooked, boiled, or drained soybeans, without salt – 970 mg.
- Cooked, boiled, or drained lima beans, without salt – 969 mg.
- Baked sweet potato – 950 mg.
- 16 Ounces Coconut Water – 900 mg.
- Low Sodium V8 – 850 mg.
- Sliced avocado – 708 mg.

- 8 Ounces Pomegranate juice – 600 mg.
- Cooked, boiled, or drained mushrooms, without salt – 555 mg.
- Sliced banana –537 mg.
- Red, ripe, raw tomatoes – 427 mg.
- Raw cantaloupe melon – 417 mg.

Table 17. Potassium–Supplement

Suggested Supplement Options	How Much and How Often
NoSalt – Potassium Chloride (640 mg per 1/4 tsp). Morton Salt Substitute – Potassium Chloride (690 mg per 1/4 tsp). NOW – Potassium Chloride Powder (365 mg per 1/8 tsp). NOW – Potassium Citrate Powder (448 mg per 1/4 tsp).	No more than 700 mg, once or twice a day with food or large smoothie. A high dosage may cause nausea. Consult with your physician, especially if intending to take twice per day. Individuals with impaired kidney function or compromised heart health should not take a potassium supplement without a doctor's approval.

Absorption Inhibitors

Alcoholic beverages and caffeine inhibit potassium absorption. More importantly, they cause your kidneys to flush additional potassium out of your system via the urine. Drinking large amounts of water will also deplete potassium due to increased urination. Low magnesium levels may increase potassium secretion from your body.

In order to bump up potassium levels in your diet, think about replacing one or two common foods (such as apples, cabbage, grapes, green beans, and plums) with foods that are rich in potassium.

Absorption Enhancers

Potassium is absorbed extremely well under most circumstances. Potassium needs magnesium to be fully utilized and to move across the cell membrane.[94]

Listen to Your Body

Low potassium can result in a variety of symptoms, such as muscle cramps, twitches, or weakness. It can also cause fatigue, low energy, abnormal heart rhythms, tingling or numbness sensations, confusion, depression, psychosis, delirium, and in some cases, hallucinations.

Excessive potassium levels (hyperkalemia) can be extremely hazardous to your health. Symptoms include muscle fatigue, weakness, paralysis, abnormal heartbeat, and cardiac arrest. Individuals with healthy kidneys rarely experience issues from consuming supplemental potassium.

Warning

When consuming adequate amounts of potassium, the human body is very efficient at managing excess via the kidneys. Nevertheless, impaired kidney function (as in diabetics) can generate dangerously high levels of potassium. It is possible for an individual to unknowingly have impaired kidney function.

Testing

Blood serum tests for potassium levels are a poor indicator of actual tissue levels. Tissue releases its stores of various nutrients in order to maintain proper levels in the blood.

A sublingual epithelial cell analysis may be considered for measuring potassium levels within your tissue. The test kit is shipped to your local physician, who collects small, soft tissue samples from the mouth. Individuals who have undergone the process state that the procedure is noninvasive and virtually painless. Tissue analysis results include levels and ratios for the following elements: magnesium, phosphorous, potassium, calcium, sodium, and chloride. You are encouraged to engage in additional research before subjecting yourself to any testing procedure.

CHAPTER THIRTEEN

Multivitamins and Minerals

Multivitamins and minerals (MVM) are compilations of vitamins, minerals, and trace elements needed to sustain physical and mental wellbeing. A quality MVM will provide additional nutrient requirements for optimal bone health, such as vitamin A and boron.

The National Institutes of Health[95] states, "Women, the elderly, people with more education, more income, healthier diets and lifestyles, and lower body weights, and people in the western United States use MVMs most often. Smokers and members of certain ethnic and racial groups (such as African Americans, Hispanics, and Native Americans) are less likely to take a daily MVM."

An editorial published by the *Annals of Internal Medicine*[96] claimed that vitamin and mineral supplements are a waste of money. I could not disagree more. Upon reading the article, certain statements caught my attention, such as:

> "Efficacy of vitamin supplements for primary prevention in community-dwelling adults with no nutritional deficiencies."
>
> "Use of a multivitamin supplement in a well-nourished elderly population did not prevent cognitive decline."

I agree with the conclusion that vitamin and mineral supplements may not benefit people who are "well-nourished" and people "with no nutritional deficiencies." Basically, if you are nutritionally whole, you won't gain added benefits from multivitamins.

The editorial resulted in the following headlines:

"Experts: Don't Waste Your Money on Multivitamins." (*WebMD*)

"Vitamins Lack Clear Health Benefits, May Pose Risks." (*Forbes*)

"Medical journal: 'Case closed' against vitamin pills." (*USA Today*)

I am deeply troubled by the message conveyed as it may persuade individuals suffering from nutritional deficiencies to avoid supplements that can improve their health. Many individuals who do suffer from nutrient deficiencies will benefit immensely from quality supplementation. The very purpose of multivitamins and other supplements is to fill in the areas where you are not nutritionally whole.

Additionally, the Harvard School of Public Health states, "Looking at all the evidence, the potential health benefits of taking a standard daily multivitamin seem to outweigh the potential risks for most people."[97] Furthermore, The Agency for Healthcare Research and Quality states,

"Multivitamin/mineral supplement use may prevent cancer in individuals with poor or suboptimal nutritional status."[98]

Specialized formulations of MVMs are recommended and sometimes prescribed for prenatal care. This is likely because a high-quality MVM is far more efficient at filling a broad spectrum of nutritional gaps. They cannot and should not be used in place of healthy food choices. They most definitely should be used to "top off" your nutritional tank when diet alone does not meet all your nutrient requirements.

I have personally witnessed the impact of a high-quality MVM on individuals who were nutrient-deficient. For example, I gave a doctor and a homeless man each a seven-day supply of MVMs. They were both amazed by the difference in how they felt. The doctor had been suffering from chronic fatigue and attributed her condition to work-related stress. Within a week of taking the MVM, she was astonished by the significant improvement in her focus and energy.

The homeless man had been suffering from a severe and frequent cough for more than a month. Within three days, he came to me extremely excited and said, "What did you give me? My cough is almost gone! I haven't felt this good in years! Thank you so much!"

The key to these and other success stories is the quality of the MVM. I introduced high-quality MVMs to individuals who had been taking extremely popular lower-grade MVMs for years. They all have expressed how much better they feel within days of switching to the products I recommended. I received no financial incentives from the manufacturers or products I recommended.

How Much and How Often

Try any high-quality MVM six days a week for up to thirty days, either in half doses or at full strength. If you do not notice results, many retailers offer full refunds. A comprehensive list of the hundred MVM products to choose from can be found at www.MultivitaminGuide.org.

Quite often, a high-quality MVM will turn your urine a vibrant yellowish hue. Don't panic. This is mainly the excess B-12 being flushed out of your system. If you are nutrient deficient, your energy and mental focus should noticeably increase in anywhere between three days and two weeks. The more nutrient deficient you are, the quicker and more noticeable the results should be. If you are prone to coughs, illness, or infections, you may experience a decrease in frequency, severity, and duration. There are many benefits that a high-quality MVM can offer individuals with mild to severe nutrient deficiencies.

High-quality MVMs cost much more than the more familiar brands. As with most things, you get what you pay for. I assign a four-tier categorization based on overall quality to MVMs. The fourth tier is the worst and the first tier is the best. Each level consists of several brands. Over the years, first-tier brand prices have dramatically decreased. They initially sold for as much as $120 for a one-month supply. They currently sell for about half of what they once did. First-tier MVM products practically work miracles.

I usually stay within the second-tier range, which used to cost around $18 for a one-month supply. However, you do have to augment them with two or three additional standalone supplements, which drives up the cost. A monthly price breakdown for recommended MVMs is contained in Chapter 14 section entitled "Product List."

First-tier and second-tier brands have an exceedingly high absorption rate. Therefore, consider taking only one third or one half of the recommended dose per day. For instance, if the manufacturer's recommendation is two pills per day, only take one. If you are a meticulous individual, you can break one tablet in half. Take one half with breakfast and the other half during lunch. Not only will you obtain the additional nutrients you need, but your supply will last twice as long, which translates into savings. Individuals who drink alcohol excessively or maintain a very poor diet may require the full recommended dose.

First-tier MVMs frequently contain an exceptionally balanced ratio of vitamins, minerals, and trace elements. Second-tier MVMs may contain extreme amounts of some vitamins. Third- and fourth-tier MVMs are of extremely poor-quality and may sell for as low as $20 for a one-year supply (approx. $1.67 per month). They use the least desirable forms of vitamins and minerals and are one step removed from a placebo. They seem to put more money into TV advertisements than the vitamins themselves. In the long run, investing in high-quality MVMs is also more cost-effective due to the potential mental and physical health benefits.

Many MVMs that are second tier and below contain one or two low-quality mineral formulations such as magnesium oxide. As previously stated, low-quality mineral formulations do not absorb well. Additionally, minerals compete for the same absorption receptors, causing some minerals to inhibit the absorption of others.

Excess nutrients from MVMs combined with a nutrient-dense diet can introduce health problems. Keep in mind that individuals who regularly take MVMs typically maintain a healthier diet than those who do not. If your diet is reasonably sound, moderate your MVM intake.

In addition, do not take an MVM every day. Four to six days per week should be more than sufficient. There is no benefit from overdosing nutrients with the short-term exception of correcting a deficiency. Doing so merely wastes money and can be detrimental to your long-term health. If your diet is nutrient-poor, taking the full recommended serving five to seven days per week may be required.

Supplements are not designed to supply all your nutritional needs. They are a means to fill nutritional gaps in your diet (see Chapter 18 "Supplement Abuse").

Table 18. Multivitamins Ratings
(MultivaminGuide.org — Top 10 of 100)[99]

Company	Product
NATURELO Premium Supplements.	Whole Food Multivitamin.
Xtend-Life Natural Products.	Total Balance.
Douglas Laboratories.	Ultra Preventive X.
USANA Health Sciences.	HealthPak.
Dr. Mercola.	Whole Food Multivitamin PLUS.
Shaklee.	Vitalizer.
Life Extension.	Life Extension Mix.
Metagenics.	Wellness Essentials.
Nutrilite (Amway).	Double X.
Garden of Life.	Vitamin Code.

View the entire list at http://www.multivitaminguide.org

Absorption Inhibitors

Absorption can be inhibited by phytate and caffeine.

Absorption Enhancers

Multivitamins/minerals are absorbed best when taken with a meal.

Best Formulation

- Xtend-Life Natural Products – Total Balance.
- Douglas Laboratories – Ultra Preventive X.
- NATURELO – Whole Food Multivitamin.
- Life Extension – Life Extension Mix.
- Life Extension – Two-Per-Day (capsule or tablet).
- Optimum Nutrition – Opti-Men/Opti-Women.

If you are currently taking an MVM found at your typical drugstore, you are encouraged to switch to a higher-quality brand. MVMs found in most drugstores seemingly spend massive amounts of money on commercials as opposed to better ingredients. This benefits their bottom line but does very little for your short- and long-term health. It is often true that something is better than nothing. However, when it comes to your health, investing in better quality MVMs can yield much greater results.

Purchase MVMs from a reputable vitamin store or directly from the manufacturer's website. Third-party websites that do not specialize in health and nutrition have spotty quality control. Some individuals have received counterfeit or expired products.

Listen to Your Body

General symptoms of a deficiency may include fatigue, insomnia, hair loss, dry skin, headache, depression, anxiety, frequent infections, and slow healing. Excess consumption may cause stomach cramps, nausea, or diarrhea.

Warning

Multivitamins can irritate your stomach, especially if not taken with a meal. Quality multivitamins contain high concentrations of nutrients. You likely only need one half of the manufacturer's suggested dose. I also encourage skipping a day (or two) periodically to purge excess from your system.

CHAPTER FOURTEEN

Daily Supplement Schedules

Daily supplement schedules have been developed according to the typical income, lifestyle, and nutritional needs of specific age groups. Proceed with caution, especially if you are taking medications, have allergies, or have an underlying health condition. You should also consider consulting with your doctor before adopting a schedule.

You will find that phosphorous, protein, and carbohydrates have not been added to the schedules. Please refer to the "How Much and How Often" section of their associated chapters for more details. Additionally, please refer to Chapter 8 "Liver & Kidney Health" for a list of foods that promote liver health.

You will also find that potassium is not included in the daily schedules. However, potassium is an important mineral for bone health. Therefore, if you elect to take supplemental potassium, please ensure that you do not exceed the manufacturer's recommended amount per serving. Consider adding potassium salt to your meals and your smoothies. High concentrations can cause ulcers and can also be fatal.

Due to a myriad of variables and factors, you may need to deviate from the schedules provided to address unique conditions. For example, the more direct sun exposure you obtain—based on your region and lifestyle—the less vitamin D supplementation you may require.

Multivitamins and Minerals (MVM)

The Life Extension Two-Per-Day MVM is the example used in the following schedules. The manufacturer's suggested dosage is two tablets per day with meals. However, only one tablet per day is recommended in the schedules.

Each schedule recommends that only half of the suggested dose be taken for the entire day for several reasons. These are high-quality vitamins for the cost, which means they contain formulations of nutrients, such as folate instead of folic acid, which will be readily absorbed and utilized in your system, so much so that your urine may emit a bright yellow, amber, or orange glow. Do not let this discoloration alarm you as it is simply your kidneys disposing of excess vitamin B.

When you purchase a better-quality multivitamin, you typically only need 50 percent or less of the manufacturer's recommended usage. You can even break a tablet in half to accomplish this, if needed. Additionally, you will receive nutrients from food, beverages, and other standalone vitamin products. The goal is to achieve balance. You are also encouraged to go one or two days per week without taking a MVM to allow your body time to metabolize or purge excess.

There are products of even higher quality. However, they are more cost prohibitive, as indicated in the *Product List* following the *Daily Supplement Schedules*. If you choose to move up to the more expensive brands, you will not need as many additional standalone products to fill in the gaps. This increases convenience and offsets some of the added cost. Even then, it is strongly recommended to only take half of their daily suggested use (with one or two exceptions).

IMPORTANT: You can take multivitamins with breakfast or lunch. I caution against taking them with your last meal as it could result in bouts of insomnia.

The "Total" Approach

When taking supplements, you should always consider the total nutrient intake and likely absorption rate. For example, Life Extension Two-Per-Day contains 1000 IU of vitamin D3 in each pill. Citracal Petites contain 250 IU of vitamin D3 in each pill. A glass of milk also contains vitamin D.

When you combine the total amount of vitamin D provided from all sources, how much more do you require from a standalone supplement? It is advisable to assume a slightly lower absorption rate for individual nutrients within multivitamins, as some will compete with others to be accepted.

This "total" approach should be applied to all vitamins and minerals obtained from food, the sun, and supplements. Train yourself not to view supplemental vitamins and minerals in a vacuum. Consider all sources.

More Schedules Are Available

The following schedules are based on the current ingredients in Life Extension Two-Per-Day multivitamins. Additional schedules are available for Book Club members through my author website: https://bryantlusk.com/sharethehealth/

Table 19. Daily Supplement Schedule Ages 60+

	Breakfast	Lunch	Dinner	Optional^
Sun.	Magnesium 100–200 mg	Iodine 150–400 mcg* Calcium 200–300 mg	Magnesium 100–200 mg Copper 2 mg	
Mon.	Multivitamin Magnesium 100–200 mg D3 2000 IU	K2 90–250 mcg Calcium 200–300 mg	Magnesium 100–200 mg Zinc 10–25 mg	Calcium 200–300 mg
Tues.	Multivitamin Magnesium 100–200 mg	K2 90–250 mcg Calcium 200–300 mg	Magnesium 100–200 mg Zinc 10–25 mg	Calcium 200–300 mg
Wed.	Multivitamin Magnesium 100–200 mg D3 2000 IU	K2 90–250 mcg Calcium 200–300 mg	Magnesium 100–200 mg	Calcium 200–300 mg
Thurs.	Multivitamin Magnesium 100–200 mg	K2 90–250 mcg Calcium 200–300 mg Iodine 150–400 mcg*	Magnesium 100–200 mg Zinc 10–25 mg	Calcium 200–300 mg
Fri.	Multivitamin Magnesium 100–200 mg D3 2000 IU	K2 90–250 mcg Calcium 200–300 mg	Magnesium 100–200 mg Zinc 10–25 mg	Calcium 200–300 mg
Sat.	Magnesium 100–200 mg		Magnesium 100–200 mg	Multi-vitamin

NOTE: *This schedule provides a comprehensive approach for individuals this age. However, the daily supplement schedule for ages 25-34 is my minimum recommendation for this age group.*

^ *Optional: can add any or all supplements listed here to your weekly schedule.*

* *Iodine above 250 mcg should be liquid nascent form.*

Table 20. Daily Supplement Schedule Ages 45–59

	Breakfast	Lunch	Dinner	Optional^
Sun.	Magnesium 100–200 mg	Iodine 100–400 mcg* Calcium 200–300 mg	Magnesium 100–200 mg	
Mon.	Multivitamin Magnesium 100–200 mg	K2 90–250 mcg Calcium 200–300 mg D3 1000–2000 IU	Magnesium 100–200 mg Zinc 10–25 mg	Calcium 200–300 mg
Tues.	Multivitamin Magnesium 100–200 mg	K2 90–250 mcg Calcium 200–300 mg	Magnesium 100–200 mg Zinc 10–25 mg	
Wed.	Multivitamin Magnesium 100–200 mg	K2 90–250 mcg Calcium 200–300 mg D3 1000–2000 IU	Magnesium 100–200 mg	Calcium 200–300 mg
Thurs.	Multivitamin Magnesium 100–200 mg	Iodine 100–400 mcg* K2 90–250 mcg Calcium 200–300 mg	Magnesium 100–200 mg Zinc 10–25 mg	
Fri.	Multivitamin Magnesium 100–200 mg	K2 90–250 mcg Calcium 200–300 mg D3 1000–2000 IU	Magnesium 100–200 mg Zinc 10–25 mg	Calcium 200–300 mg
Sat.	Magnesium 100–200 mg		Magnesium 100–200 mg	Multi-vitamin

NOTE: This schedule provides a comprehensive approach for individuals this age. However, the daily supplement schedule for ages 25-34 is my minimum recommendation for this age group.

^ Optional: can add any or all supplements listed here to your weekly schedule.

* Iodine above 250 mcg should be liquid nascent form.

Table 21. Daily Supplement Schedule Ages 35–44

	Breakfast	Lunch	Dinner	Optional^
Sun.	Iodine 100–400 mcg*		Magnesium 100–200 mg	
Mon.	Multivitamin Magnesium 100–200 mg	K2 90–250 mcg Calcium 200–300 mg	Magnesium 100–200 mg Zinc 10–25 mg	
Tues.	Multivitamin D3 1000–2000 IU	K2 90–250 mcg Calcium 200–300 mg	Magnesium 100–200 mg	
Wed.	Multivitamin Magnesium 100–200 mg	K2 90–250 mcg Calcium 200–300 mg	Magnesium 100–200 mg Zinc 10–25 mg	
Thurs.	Multivitamin D3 1000–2000 IU	K2 90–250 mcg Calcium 200–300 mg	Magnesium 100–200 mg	Iodine 100–400 mcg*
Fri.	Multivitamin Magnesium 100–200 mg	K2 90–250 mcg Calcium 200–300 mg	Magnesium 100–200 mg Zinc 10–25 mg	
Sat.	D3 1000–2000 IU	Calcium 200–300 mg	Magnesium 100–200 mg	Multi-vitamin

NOTE: This schedule provides a comprehensive approach for individuals this age. However, the daily supplement schedule for ages 25-34 is my minimum recommendation for this age group.

^ Optional: can add any or all supplements listed here to your weekly schedule.

* Iodine above 250 mcg should be liquid nascent form.

Table 22. Daily Supplement Schedule Ages 25–34

	Breakfast	Lunch	Optional^
Sun.			
Mon.	Multivitamin Magnesium 100–200 mg D3 1000–2000 IU	Calcium 200–300 mg K2 90–250 mcg	Iodine 100–400 mcg*
Tues.	Multivitamin Magnesium 100–200 mg	Calcium 200–300 mg	Zinc 10–25 mg
Wed.	Multivitamin Magnesium 100–200 mg D3 1000–2000 IU	Calcium 200–300 mg K2 90–250 mcg	
Thurs.	Multivitamin Magnesium 100–200 mg Iodine 100–400 mcg*	Calcium 200–300 mg	Zinc 10–25 mg
Fri.	Multivitamin Magnesium 100–200 mg D3 1000–2000 IU	Calcium 200–300 mg K2 90–250 mcg	
Sat.	Magnesium 100–200 mg	Calcium 200–300 mg	Zinc 10–25 mg Multivitamin

^ Optional: can add any or all supplements listed here to your weekly schedule.

* Iodine above 250 mcg should be liquid nascent form.

Table 23. Daily Supplement Schedule Ages 18–24

	Breakfast or Lunch	Optional but Recommended^
Sun.		
Mon.	Multivitamin Magnesium 100–200 mg	D3 1000–2000 IU
Tues.	Multivitamin Magnesium 100–200 mg	Iodine 100–400 mcg*
Wed.	Multivitamin Magnesium 100–200 mg	D3 1000–2000 IU
Thurs.	Multivitamin Magnesium 100–200 mg	
Fri.	Multivitamin Magnesium 100–200 mg	D3 1000–2000 IU
Sat.		Multivitamin

^ Optional: can add any or all supplements listed here to your weekly schedule.

* Iodine above 250 mcg should be liquid nascent form.

Product List

Several products and manufacturers were discussed in each chapter. Below is a consolidated list. Although these are brands I have come to trust, you may find others more to your liking.

As mentioned previously, purchase your products from an actual vitamin store or directly from the manufacturer's website. Otherwise, be vigilant when buying vitamins through third-party internet retailers. The problem is not with the retailer; rather, there are issues with some of the sellers who use them.

It is worth repeating that there have been instances of sellers shipping counterfeit products. There have also been instances of sellers shipping expired or nearly expired products. This does not happen often, but it does warrant concern. Make certain to read the reviews for the seller. Examine the product and the expiration date. Some sellers have even stooped to covering expiration dates with barcode labels. Do not become frightened, but do be careful.

Magnesium

Form:

- Magnesium glycinate (calming effect that may aid sleep).
- Magnesium citrate.
- Magnesium aspartate.
- Magnesium taurate.

Product:

- Swanson – Chelated Magnesium Bisglycinate (133 mg).
- Whole Foods 365 – Magnesium Glycinate (~133 mg).
- Now Foods – Magnesium Citrate (200 mg).
- Good State – Ionic (liquid) Magnesium (100 mg).
- Doctor's Best – Chelated Magnesium Glycinate (100 mg).

Vitamin K2

Form:

- Menaquinone – 7 (MK-7).

Product:

- Jarrow Formulas – MK-7 (90 mcg).
- Sports Research – MK-7 (100 mcg).
- Nutrigold – MK-7 (100 mcg).
- Now Foods – MK-7 (100 mcg).

Zinc

Form:

- Zinc orotate (absorbs exceptionally well).
- Zinc monomethionine (absorbs extremely well).
- Zinc picolinate (absorbs extremely well; may irritate empty stomach).
- Zinc citrate (absorbs well; may irritate empty stomach).
- Zinc gluconate (absorbs well; may irritate empty stomach).

Product:

- Jarrow Formulas – Zinc Balance: Zinc (15 mg) Copper (1 mg).
- Swanson – Zinc Orotate (10 mg).
- Whole Foods 365 – Zinc (15 mg) Copper (1 mg).
- Solgar – Zinc Picolinate: (22 mg).
- Pure Encapsulations – Zinc 30: Zinc Picolinate (30 mg) (high dose, take less frequently).
- Kal – Zinc Orotate (30 mg) (high dose, take less frequently).
- Liquid ionic zinc (various brands) (15 mg).

Vitamin D

Form:

- D3.

Product:

- Life Extension – D3 (1,000 IU).
- Nutrigold – D3 (2,000 IU).
- Sports Research – D3 (2,000 IU).

Calcium

Form:

- Calcium citrate (absorbs well with or without food).
- Calcium carbonate (take with food).

Product:

- Citracal Petites – Calcium Citrate (200 mg) D3 (250 IU).
- Pure Encapsulations – Calcium Citrate (150 mg).
- Bluebonnet – Calcium Citrate (250 mg) D3 (200 IU) Mag. Aspartate (100 mg).
- NATURELO – Plant-Based Calcium (150 mg) D3 (6.25 mcg) Mag. Glycinate (50 mg).

Iodine

Form:

- Nascent (atomic) iodine (absorbs exceptionally well; superior form of iodine).
- Molecular iodine (absorbs well on an empty stomach).
- Potassium iodide (absorbs moderately well).

Product:

- LL – Magnetic Clay Nascent Iodine – 1 oz (400 mcg per drop).
- Go Nutrients – Iodine Edge Nascent Iodine (~300 mcg per drop).
- NOW – Kelp Caps (150 mcg).

Potassium

Form:

- Potassium Chloride.
- Potassium Citrate.

Product:

- NoSalt – Potassium Chloride (640 mg per 1/4 tsp).
- Morton Salt Substitute – Potassium Chloride (690 mg per 1/4 tsp).
- NOW – Potassium Chloride Powder (365 mg per 1/8 tsp).
- NOW – Potassium Citrate Powder (448 mg per 1/4 tsp).

Multivitamin

Product (estimated cost* at half dose usage):

- Xtend-Life Natural Products – Total Balance ($26/month).
- Douglas Laboratories – Ultra Preventive X ($43/month).
- NATURELO – Whole Food Multivitamin ($45/month full dose).
- Life Extension – Life Extension Mix ($30/month).
- Life Extension – Two-Per-Day ($5/month). **
- Optimum Nutrition – Opti-Men/Opti-Women ($5/month). **

* estimated cost as of February 3, 2019

** additional cost required due to need for more standalone vitamins

CHAPTER FIFTEEN

Protein

Impacts: Bone Density, Immune System, Mental Health, Heart Health, Healing, Hair Health

Protein is one of the body's most utilized sources for building skeletal muscle and soft tissue, and for brain function. Inadequate protein intake is extremely unhealthy and can lead to growth retardation (in children), reduction in muscle mass, poor bone structure, decreased immunity, heart issues, and more. Elderly men who exhibit protein deficiency have higher incidents of osteoporotic fracture (SOF).[100,101]

Adequate protein intake is necessary for healthy bones. However, some studies suggest a correlation between excessive protein intake and bone loss. Excessive protein can also be unhealthy for individuals with impaired liver or kidney function. Excessive protein can raise blood sugar, cause unwanted weight gain, place unwanted stress on your kidneys, and weaken your bones by leaching calcium from them. Moreover, excessive protein can promote cancer cell growth.

Excessive protein coupled with low mineral intake can lower serum pH, resulting in acidosis. The body reacts to acidosis by releasing calcium from the bones to regain the proper pH balance, resulting in less-than-optimal bone density. You can counteract some of the acidic effects of excess protein with fruits and dark green vegetables. Also, ensure you are obtaining adequate (not excessive) magnesium, potassium, and calcium to maintain the balance. The body only needs the amount of protein it needs. Consuming more will not make your body need or utilize more. Balance is key.

With animal-based proteins, research indicates a direct correlation between heavy red meat consumption and an increased risk of cardiovascular disease (CVD) and cancer mortality.[102] Red meat cooking methods may be more of a factor than the meat itself.

Weight-based protein calculators:

- https://www.calculatorpro.com/calculator/protein-calculator
- https://www.bodybuilding.com/fun/calpro.htm

Excessive protein intake for workout enthusiasts is not beneficial to muscle gain. In fact, it can prevent you from reaching your fitness goals. You should only consume the amount of protein required to maintain your health and achieve your fitness goals. More is not better. Anything your body cannot process becomes waste.

Vegetarians

Vegetarians can get enough basic protein via plants. However, important amino acids, such as L-taurine and L-lysine, are only abundant in animal-based protein. L-lysine is one of nine essential amino acids that cannot be manufactured by your body. The good news is that L-taurine and L-lysine can be supplemented.

How Much and How Often

Overall daily protein intake for a moderately active person should fall between 0.35 g and 0.45 g of protein per pound of bodyweight. Those undertaking advanced exercise regimens will likely require higher protein intake, possibly in the range of 0.4 to 0.65 g per pound of bodyweight. Professional athlete requirements are even higher. In case you were wondering, heavy lifting at the local gym does not come anywhere near a professional athlete's exercise regimen.

Beverages such as milk contain protein and carbohydrates. If using protein powders with milk or juice, add the number of milligrams (mg) listed on the milk or juice label with the amount contained in the powder you are adding. If your objective is to consume 25 g of protein in one serving, be mindful that a serving of milk contains 8 g. Therefore, you only need to add an additional 17 g of protein powder to achieve 25 g of protein in total.

Weight training in moderation builds strong bones and helps prevent osteoporosis. It stimulates osteoblasts and osteocalcin production. Excessive exercise can damage your joints over time.

A balanced approach will also provide your muscles, tendons, bones, and joints better protection from injury, and will allow for faster recovery.

Table 24. Protein–Food

Food Type and Quantity	How Often
tuna, chicken, turkey, bison, lean beef or pork, wild salmon, tilapia, white fish, cage-free eggs, milk, cheese (dairy), beans, seeds, nuts, nut butter.	One serving of any of these items 2 or 3 times a day.

Table 25. Protein–Supplement

Suggested Supplement Options	How Much and How Often
Optimum Nutrition – Whey Protein Isolate Powder (or any reputable manufacturer). Blackberries, blueberries, and acacia powder are excellent sources of fiber to include with your protein. Mixing with organic milk provides additional calcium.	0.1 to 0.2 grams per pound of body weight every other day or as needed. 0.15 to 0.25 grams per pound of body weight for advanced exercise regimens. Supplemental protein should NOT provide the bulk of your daily requirement.

Absorption Inhibitors

Protein absorption is rarely inhibited within a healthy GI tract.

Absorption Enhancers

Papaya, cheeses, and certain vegetables provide digestive enzymes to more effectively break down protein-rich meals.

Best Formulation

- Whey isolate protein powder (absorbs exceptionally well)
- Optimum Nutrition's Whey Protein Powder contains 24 g of protein, 5.5 g of branched-chain amino acids (BCAAs), and 4 g of glutamine per serving. It is loaded with whey protein isolates, which absorb exceptionally well.

Listen to Your Body

Symptoms of protein deficiency include: skin discoloration, skin rashes, lethargy, fatigue, difficulty sleeping, excessive sleeping (lack of energy), muscle weakness, muscle loss, frequent infections, slow wound healing, hair loss, brittle hair, mood swings, depression, anxiety, and apathy. Excessive protein may present itself as low calcium, gout, or kidney stones.

Warning

Excessive protein intake may trigger your body to release calcium from your bones. Also, there are some health risks associated with excessive protein intake, especially for individuals with impaired kidney or liver function. Additional risks may be present because of cancer-promoting agents found in some protein sources, or introduced by food preparation.

CHAPTER SIXTEEN

Carbohydrates

Impacts: Energy, Weight Loss, Bone Health, Heart Health, Brain Health

Healthy carbohydrates are the body's best sources of fuel for physical endurance, brain activity, and exercise for strong muscles and bones. Not all carbs are created equal. Carbohydrates derived from bananas, berries, beans, chickpeas, yams, wild rice, and organic milk have a much healthier impact than those from cookies, doughnuts, potato chips, and soda.

Healthy carbohydrates provide several important nutrients and allow for the stable release of glucose for adenosine triphosphate (ATP) energy. In addition, some forms of healthy carbs are high in fiber, which is critical to sustained food absorption and weight management. Individuals with high intakes of dietary fiber are at significantly lower risk of developing coronary heart disease, stroke, diabetes, obesity, hypertension, and other diseases. A moderately active person should consume 0.7–1.0 g of healthy carbohydrates per pound of body weight a day. Contrary to misinformation from faux diets, healthy carbs can be very beneficial to weight management and brain energy.

Studies associate reduced fatigue and improved exercise performance with multiple transportable carbohydrates rather than a single carbohydrate.[103] Exercise is integral to bone health and the prevention of osteoporosis.

Contrary to certain diet fads, carbohydrate-rich foods (not processed) provide a readily available source of fuel for muscle glycogen synthesis and can be very beneficial in workout recovery meals. Moderate workouts make bones stronger and more durable. Moreover, low potassium is likely the reason many people have difficulty with metabolizing carbohydrates. Low potassium weakens your bones and adversely impacts many vital functions, such as heart rhythm and insulin resistance. **Here again, diet-fad enthusiasts view carbohydrates as a problem to eliminate, versus a symptom of a far more detrimental health issue**.

Excessive simple carbohydrate consumption can be harmful to your health. However, a balanced intake of healthy carbohydrates is very beneficial.

Healthy Carbohydrate Options

- Sweet Potatoes
- Blueberries
- Oatmeal (High-Fiber)
- Acorn Squash
- Barley
- Buckwheat
- Brown Rice
- Quinoa

Beyond Nutrition

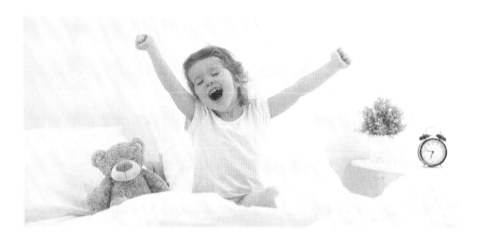

Sleep

Chronic sleep deprivation (CSD) has been demonstrated to significantly diminish 25(OH)D (vitamin D) levels and bone mineral density (BMD).[104,105,106] Individuals age 18–60 should obtain at least seven hours of sleep per night. Individuals age 61–64 should obtain 7–9 hours of sleep. Individuals that are age 65 and older should obtain 7–8 hours of sleep. Moreover, the quality of sleep is just as important as the duration.

Seven to 8 hours of undisturbed sleep appears to be the healthiest duration of sleep for many adults. Sleep studies[107] have identified a possible correlation between increased incidence of natural death and sleep intervals that are less than seven hours.

According to the CDC:[108]

> "Insufficient sleep is associated with a number of chronic diseases and conditions—such as diabetes, cardiovascular disease, obesity, and depression—which threaten our nation's health. Notably, insufficient sleep is associated with the onset of these diseases and also poses important implications for their management and outcome."

400–600 mg of calcium and 400 mg of magnesium taken daily (but not together) is a natural cure for some forms of insomnia.

Chamomile tea also contains relaxing agents that can help individuals to go to sleep. I caution against sleep aids such as melatonin unless used very sparingly. Individuals over sixty years of age may need supplemental melatonin as their bodies tend to produce less than nominal amounts. Calcium naturally increases your body's melatonin production.[109]

Exercise

Resistance training forces your bones and muscles to adapt and grow denser. Younger and middle-age adults are encouraged to make time to exercise for 30-45 minutes a day, 4-5 days a week. Taking a full week off every fifth or sixth week will make you stronger. Ensure that you follow the supplement schedule for your age group for better results. Using proper posture and technique will yield far greater results than tossing extremely heavy weights into the air.

Individuals 65 and older (with exceptions, of course, depending on fitness level of and health) should consider exercising 20-30 minutes a day, 4-5 days a week. Stretch bands, light dumbbells, and body-weight exercise may be more to your liking. There is also a weighted vest one can wear while enjoying a walk. Always ensure that you wear comfortable shoes that will not easily slip. According to the International Osteoporosis Foundation:

> "Several exercises are not suitable for people with osteoporosis as they can exert strong force on relatively weak bone. Dynamic abdominal exercises like sit-ups and excessive trunk flexion can cause vertebral crush fractures. Twisting movements such as a golf swing can also cause fractures. Exercises that involve abrupt or explosive loading, or high-impact loading, are also contraindicated. Daily activities such as bending to pick up objects can cause vertebral fracture and should be avoided."[110]

Feet

As with the liver and kidneys, here lies another subject that is rarely discussed in conjunction with bone health. Your skeletal alignment begins with your feet. A foot injury or abnormality can impact your cadence, gait, alignment, joints, posture and level of activity. Improperly-sized footwear, or footwear that does not adequately support the foot can gradually induce unnecessary wear and tear on your bones, spine, joints, and nerves.

Morton's Neuroma

You are encouraged to invest in orthopedic sandals and slippers that not only support your arch, but also decompresses the nerves that travel between the bones of the toes. Shoes that squeeze the sides of your foot can irritate nerves that run through the ball of your foot, and between the bones of your toes. Pain in the ball of the foot may be caused by longstanding irritation of those nerves. This can then result in a common foot condition called Morton's neuroma: a swollen and inflamed nerve.

Eventually, if left untreated, the condition worsens to the point where an individual unconsciously becomes more sedentary. A sedentary lifestyle places you at much greater risk of developing osteopenia and osteoporosis. Surgery to correct the condition is the final solution: however, there are steps you can take before getting to that point.

Really good orthotic house shoes (slippers), sandals, and inserts not only support the arch, but they also have a rise (bump) just behind the ball of the foot to laterally (side-to-side) spread the bones apart and remove pressure from the nerve. They can be a lot more expensive than drugstore brands, but you will likely be amazed at the difference over time. I suggest searching the internet with the phrase "best orthotics for Morton's neuroma."

When I became aware of this condition, I gave away twelve pairs of shoes (average cost $200 each) and restocked my closet with the next size up. I also invested in a few pairs of costly shoe inserts. My feet haven't felt this good in over a decade and my military posture has reemerged.

Proper realignment of the foot can relieve a variety of skeletal aches and pains, from the bottom of the foot all of the way up to the base of the skull. Improved alignment spreads weight more evenly across your bones and joints. Moreover, your posture will also benefit. Many individuals wear shoes that are too small, thereby placing enormous pressure on the bones and nerves in their feet. Proper footwear can work wonders for everyone and their skeletal health.

Plantar Fasciitis

Plantar fasciitis is another common foot injury that can be extremely debilitating. It is often recognized as a sharp pain at the base of the heel. Footwear that does not support the arch properly places you at greater risk of developing this injury. In turn, the pain can be so excruciating when walking that you choose to become sedentary to avoid it. Over time, this aversion to walking can lead to less than optimal bone density.

As with Morton's neuroma, plantar fasciitis will adversely impact your natural gait, cadence, and posture. In doing so your bones and joints will suffer from unnatural motion and pressure points. The human body is a system. Nothing inside of it occurs in a vacuum. There is always the potential for ripple effects to be considered.

Feet are the foundation for the entire skeletal structure. Therefore, we must always consider long-term health when purchasing footwear. Footwear should not be overly snug. This will help prevent Morton's neuroma. Moreover, one should always purchase footwear (or inserts) with strong arch support.

Prescription Drugs for Osteoporosis

Certain drugs may be prescribed to address bone loss. Some studies suggest a link between certain osteoporosis prescription drugs and cancer; however, I have not conducted enough research into this topic to offer a worthwhile opinion as it is outside the scope of vitamin therapy.

Drugs that have been used include:

- Bisphosphonates (Fosamax, Boniva, Actonel, and Reclast).
- Calcitonin (Fortical and Miacalcin).
- Hormone therapy or estrogen.
- SERMS (selective estrogen receptor modulators) (Evista or raloxifene).
- Parathyroid hormone (Forteo or teriparatide).
- Prolia biologic.

There is growing concern over the potential long-term adverse effects of some, if not all, of the above drugs. Discuss any concerns you may have with your physician prior to accepting a prescription. If you choose to conduct your own research, do so without prejudice. Moreover, always consider the source of the information.

CHAPTER EIGHTEEN

Supplement Abuse

According to *Merriam-Webster*,[111] a supplement is "something that is added to something else in order to make it complete." Unfortunately, some people have convinced themselves and others that their bodies function better with excessive supplementation instead of a balanced ratio.

For example, excessive calcium intake has been associated with increased incidents of cancer, heart disease, sudden cardiac arrest, and stroke. The goal is not to exceed intake, but rather to optimize calcium utilization and bone health.

As discussed previously, iodine supplement abuse appears to be on the rise. Although the RDA for iodine is only 150 mcg (micrograms) per day, individuals have suggested daily supplementation as high as 12.5 mg (milligrams) a day. This is more than 83 times the RDA. As stated in Chapter 11, the belief that people in Japan consume 13.8 mg of iodine a day may have resulted from an incorrectly applied equation used on a research paper written in 1967.

As of 2004, average iodine intake in the United States ranged from 138 mcg to 353 mcg (micrograms) per day.[112] Based on these actual intake levels, if 12.5 mg (milligrams) of daily iodine were required to maintain thyroid health (as is suggested by mega-dosers) one would expect the majority of the US population to develop goiter and other dramatic health issues associated with severe iodine deficiency. In addition, early-stage brain development would be severely impaired in newborns. To imply that people are severely iodine deficient without displaying known, associated symptoms is very problematic to say the least, and extremely misleading. However, it is possible that we need to consume a little more iodine than the RDA due to environmental factors, such as elevated fluoride and bromide intake in industrialized countries.

Moreover, how much you consume of any vitamin or mineral is not always indicative of how much you absorb. For instance, your body will absorb far more magnesium from 200 mg of chelated magnesium glycinate than it will from 200 mg of magnesium oxide. Mega-dosers often fail to differentiate between formulations that barely absorb into your system, and those that absorb extremely well.

Individuals who mega-dose without medical supervision:

- May not have their kidneys or liver periodically tested for stress or damage.
- Likely mega-dose on multiple supplements.
- May base their decision to mega-dose on one-off studies, speculation, misinformation, or current fads.
- May not be aware that articles supporting mega-dosing on a specific supplement, often rely on very few sources versus multiple credible, independent studies.

- Ignore the compilation of scientific studies conducted in multiple countries that draw similar conclusions regarding adequate levels required for health.
- Appear to ignore the amount of nutrients they are naturally obtaining from food and beverages.

Balance Works Better

When used properly, supplements can be very effective at maintaining one's health and performance. In general, people who take supplements make healthier food choices. Hence, individuals with healthier diets require lower doses of supplemental nutrients than those who maintain a less healthy diet. Mega-dosing on supplements can undermine one's investment in healthy lifestyle choices.

The human body is an extremely complex biological machine. Nutrients are like the fuel/air/spark mixture in your car's engine—too much or too little of any one ingredient will make your engine run poorly, create more toxins, produce less energy, and shorten its life. Cells require the right amount of oxygen, fluids, vitamins, minerals, and micro-nutrients to operate at their peak. Overwhelming them with supplements may give you a short-term boost but, unfortunately, it may also diminish other vital functions and even shorten your life.

I am a strong advocate for filling nutritional holes via supplementation. I stand firmly against those who encourage abusing supplements to achieve a singular result.

Conclusion

Nutrients affect every aspect of your health, including bone health. The state of your health affects every aspect of your life. Every few years, a new wonder-diet goes viral and multitudes of "experts" flood the internet with blogs and forums telling the world that this is the diet or the superfood we have all been searching for (until the next one comes along). They also blame entire food groups for all that ails mankind in order to push their agenda. Unfortunately, they focused so heavily on quick fixes to weight loss that bone health was not factored into the equation. Their recommended diet fad may have compromised bone density in many unsuspecting individuals.

There are no miracle pills or miracle foods for long-term health. In addition, there is no such thing as the perfect diet. Regardless of the dietary path you choose, optimum bone health and performance begins at the cellular level. Give your cells and hormones the proper balance of nutrients they need to flourish; in turn, they will optimize your musculoskeletal strength throughout your life. We are all complex and unique organisms. Your cells need the right combination of tools and raw materials to construct and maintain that complex and unique structure that is "you."

The focus of this information has not been on extreme measures or dramatic lifestyle changes. The focus is on basic, key nutrient consumption to prevent or mitigate osteoporosis, low bone quality, and other health-related issues. Genetics are something we have little control over. At best, we can avoid things that mutate our DNA or aggravate genetic conditions. However, runners, weightlifters, cyclists, and couch potatoes alike can improve their bone density and quality by reversing nutrient deficiencies, removing nutrient excess, and maintaining a healthy liver. Nutrient balance obtained via vitamin therapy can also reduce dependency on costly prescription drugs. The information contained here has worked wonders for myself, my loved ones, and my colleagues. Now, it can work for you.

You will find more information regarding osteoporosis and osteopenia beyond these pages, but the material you have just read addresses several of the most commonly overlooked or misdiagnosed vitamin deficiencies in industrialized nations. Resolving them affords you the biggest health gains for the smallest investments. You do not have to start running marathons—you only have to ingest a few pills or add a few foods to your diet. That said, running marathons can be an interesting challenge and a lot of fun!

I encourage you to consider testing the information contained here. If you need supplementation to meet your nutrient requirements, consider purchasing three, seven-day pill containers. Buy different colors for morning, noon, and evening. Prefill all three with supplements each week. Be creative. Stagger your supplements in a manner that fits your eating schedule. Remember, skipping a day or two with most supplements can be beneficial.

This is your opportunity to improve your health and performance at the cellular level. This is your opportunity to offer your cells the environment they need to build and maintain an even stronger and healthier you.

Give yourself the gift of optimal bone health. Be patient. Be consistent. Be cheerful. Most importantly, be well!

SHARE THE HEALTH

Please help others who may find some of this information helpful by sharing a few words via a review on Amazon or wherever you purchase this book. It does not have to be long or detailed.

I am always hunting for information on new or improved supplement formulations, clinical studies (USA and abroad), medical journals (USA and abroad), and product reviews. Every now and then, I find a diamond in the rough. Join my *Share The Health* mailing list to receive this information. Additionally, you will be made aware of my upcoming books and associated discount offers. For more details visit:

https://bryantlusk.com/sharethehealth/

Useful Terms

Adequate Intake (AI) levels are established when there is not enough documented evidence to develop an RDA. AI is set at a level assumed to ensure nutritional adequacy. AI is based on observed intakes of the nutrient by a group of healthy persons.

Bioavailability is a term used to identify the ease or difficulty by which a nutrient is absorbed into your system. A high bioavailability means your body will readily absorb more of the nutrient.

Buffering a substance reduces its potential to irritate your digestive system through symptoms such as nausea or diarrhea. Buffering will make a substance either less alkaline or less acidic.

Chelation is a method of binding a substance to a protein to increase its bioavailability. Binding a substance to a protein greatly increases its absorption rate.

Dietary reference intakes (DRIs) are based on multiple reference values: Adequate Intake (AI), Recommended Dietary Allowance (RDA), Tolerable Upper Intake Level (UL).

Estimated Average Requirement (EAR) is the amount of a nutrient that is estimated to meet the requirement of half of all healthy individuals in the population.

Gastrointestinal (GI) Transit Time is the amount of time required for food to pass through to your stool, which is 1.5–3 days on average. High-protein meals travel at a slower pace, allowing the protein to be absorbed more fully. The foods you eat are not expelled in the same order that you eat them. Some food elements are pushed past others.

Minerals serve a multitude of functions, are used to build strong bones and teeth, regulate fluid inside and outside cells, create energy, and transfer electrical signals through your nervous system. Minerals that our bodies utilize are listed below.

Calcium, chloride, chromium, copper, fluoride, iodine, iron, magnesium, manganese, molybdenum, phosphorus, potassium, selenium, sodium, sulfur, & zinc.

Recommended Dietary Allowance (RDA) is the daily level of intake sufficient to meet the nutrient requirements of nearly all (97–98 percent) healthy individuals. The RDA is often set at the lower end of the full range of what individuals can tolerate before a nutrient becomes unsafe.

Tolerable Upper Intake Level (UL) is the maximum daily intake unlikely to cause harm.

Vitamins (Fat-Soluble) are ingested from animal fats, butter, vegetable oils, dairy, fish, and liver. The human body is very effective at storing these vitamins in your liver and fatty tissues for future use. If you regularly consume more than you need (mega-dose), some fat-soluble vitamins can damage your organs, nervous system, and brain. Fat-soluble vitamins remain available even after foods containing them are cooked. They absorb best with meals containing healthy fats (e.g., flaxseed, olive oil, eggs, avocados, lake herring, lake trout, mackerel, wild salmon, sardines, and tuna).

Fat-soluble vitamins are vitamins A, D, E, and K.

Vitamins (Water-Soluble) are mainly sourced from fruits, vegetables, and grains and are not as resilient to heat as fat-soluble vitamins. Water-soluble vitamins are not stored for very long and need to be replenished more frequently. Excess is primarily excreted via your urine.

Water-soluble vitamins are vitamins C, biotin, B1 (thiamine), B2 (riboflavin), B6 (pyridoxine), niacin (nicotinic acid), B12, folic acid, and pantothenic acid.

About Bryant Lusk

Bryant Lusk is a military veteran and author who grew up on the notorious south side of Chicago. Despite the ever-present challenges of gang violence and poverty, he became a successful Safety Inspector and Quality Control Specialist with the United States Government.

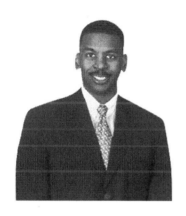

Bryant spent four years in the United States Air Force, gaining valuable experience and learning the true meaning of pride and empowerment. His desire to serve and protect others led him to write the initial installment of his *Share the Health* book series. With a determination to prevent and treat debilitating conditions, Bryant's books have helped many.

With this latest offering, Bryant shifts the focus to naturally treating osteoporosis and osteopenia, a musculoskeletal disease that inflicts back pain and bone fractures on millions of women and men worldwide. By identifying the best formulations of vitamins and minerals required to treat osteoporosis and osteopenia naturally, his approach to vitamin therapy is both affordable and effective.

Bryant enjoys learning through cultural encounters and watching classic films. He particularly enjoys spending quality time with friends and loved ones, and of course, carrying out research and writing on the things that go toward helping millions of people to improve their health and quality of life.

"I measure success by the number of people that I affect in a positive and meaningful way."

— Bryant Lusk

NOTES

[1] The Surgeon General's Report on Bone Health and Osteoporosis: What It Means to You (Last Reviewed 2017-02) https://www.bones.nih.gov/health-info/bone/SGR/surgeon-generals-report.

[2] Wheeless' Textbook of Orthopaedics. Bone Remodeling (Last Updated 2011 Sep). http://www.wheelessonline.com/ortho/bone_remodeling.

[3] International Osteoporosis Foundation. (Jan 08, 2019) Osteoporosis – Incidence and Burden https://www.iofbonehealth.org/facts-statistics.

[4] Johnell O and Kanis JA (2006) An estimate of the worldwide prevalence and disability associated with osteoporotic fractures. Osteoporosis Int. 17:1726.

[5] Arias E. United States life tables, 2009. National vital statistics reports; vol. 62, no 7. National Center for Health Statistics. 2014.

[6] National Institute of Arthritis and Musculoskeletal and Skin Diseases (Last Reviewed 2015-04) What People with Asthma Need to Know About Osteoporosis. NIH Pub. No. 16-7896.

[7] Swaminathan R. Magnesium metabolism and its disorders. Clin Biochem Rev. 2003;24(2):47–66.

[8] Saris NE, Mervaala E, Karppanen H, Khawaja JA, Lewenstam A. Magnesium. An update on physiological, clinical and analytical aspects. Clin Chim Acta. 2000;294:1–26.

[9] Fox C, Ramsoomair D, Carter C. Magnesium: its proven and potential clinical significance. South Med J. 2001;94:1195–1201.

[10] Swaminathan R. Magnesium metabolism and its disorders. Clin Biochem Rev. 2003;24(2):47–66.

[11] Shechter M, Hod H, Marks N, Behar S, Kaplinsky E, Rabinowitz B. Beneficial effect of Magnesium sulfate in acute myocardial infarction. Am J Cardiol. 1990;66:271–274. doi: 10.1016/0002-9149(90)90834-.

[12] Gu WJ, WU ZJ, WANG PF, AUNG LH, YIN RX. Intravenous magnesium prevents atrial fibrillation after coronary artery bypass grafting: a meta-analysis of 7 double-blind, placebo-controlled, randomized clinical trials. Trials. 2012;13:41. doi: 10.1186/1745-6215-13-41.

[13] ANGUS M, ANGUS Z. Cardiovascular actions of magnesium. Crit Care Clin. 2001;53:299–307.

[14] Haigney MC, Silver B, Tanglao E, et al. (1995 Oct 15) Noninvasive Measurement of Tissue Magnesium and Correlation with Cardiac Levels. Circulation. 92(8):2190-7.

[15] Burton B. Silver, Ph.D. copyright 1980–2014 Non-invasive Intracellular Mineral-Electrolyte Analysis; Published Research and References, http://www.exatest.com/Research.htm.

NOTES

[16] Brian K. Hall (2015) Bones and Cartilage – Developmental and Evolutionary Skeletal Biology (2nd Edition) https://www.sciencedirect.com/book/9780124166783/bones-and-cartilage.

[17] Editor(s): William J. Marshall, Marta Lapsley, Andrew P. Day, Ruth M. Ayling, (2014) Clinical Biochemistry: Metabolic and Clinical Aspects (3rd Edition).

[18] Clarke B. (2008 Nov) Normal Bone Anatomy and Physiology. *Clinical Journal of American Society of Nephrology.* doi: 10.2215/CJN.04151206

[19] Kwi Young Kang, In Je Kim, Sung-Hwan Park, Yeon Sik Hong (2018 March 09) Associations between trabecular bone score and vertebral fractures in patients with axial spondyloarthritis Rheumatology, Volume 57, Issue 6, 1 June 2018, Pages 1033–1040, https://doi.org/10.1093/rheumatology/key027.

[20] Hans D., Goertzen A. L., Krieg M. A., et al. (2011). "Bone microarchitecture assessed by TBS predicts osteoporotic fractures independent of bone density: The manitoba study". Journal of Bone and Mineral Research. 26 (11): 2762–9. doi:10.1002/jbmr.499. PMID 21887701.

[21] Pothuaud L., Barthe N., Krieg M., et al. (2009). "Evaluation of the Potential Use of Trabecular Bone Score to Complement Bone Mineral Density in the Diagnosis of Osteoporosis: A Preliminary spine BMD–Matched, Case-Control Study". Journal of Clinical Densitometry. 12 (2): 170–6. doi:10.1016/j.jocd.2008.11.006. PMID 19181553.

[22] Rude R.K., Singer F.R., Gruber H.E. Skeletal and hormonal effects of magnesium deficiency. J. Am. Coll.Nutr. 2009;28:131–141. doi: 10.1080/07315724.2009.10719764.

[23] Creedon A., Flynn A., Cashman K. The effect of moderately and severely restricted dietary magnesium intakes on bone composition and bone metabolism in the rat. Br. J. Nutr. 1999;82:63–71.

[24] Leidi, M.; Dellera, F.; Mariotti, M.; Banfi, G.; Crapanzano, C.; Albisetti, W.; Maier, J.A. Nitric oxide mediates low magnesium inhibition of osteoblast-like cell proliferation. J. Nutr. Biochem. 2012, 23, 1224–1229.

[25] Belluci, M.M.; Schoenmaker, T.; Rossa-Junior, C.; Orrico, S.R.; de Vries, T.J.; Everts, V. Magnesium deficiency results in an increased formation of osteoclasts. J. Nutr. Biochem. 2013, doi: 10.1016/j.jnutbio.2012.12.008.

[26] Mutlu M, Argun M, Kilic E, Saraymen R, Yazar S. Magnesium, zinc and copper status in osteoporotic, osteopenic and normal post-menopausal women. J Int Med Res 2007;35:692-5.

[27] Aydin H, Deyneli O, Yavuz D, Gözü H, Mutlu N, Kaygusuz I, Akalin S. Short-term oral magnesium supplementation suppresses bone turnover in postmenopausal osteoporotic women. Biol Trace Elem Res 2010;133:136-43.

NOTES

[28] Ko HJ, Youn CH, Kim HM, et al. (2014 Jun) Dietary Magnesium Intake and Risk of Cancer: A Meta-Analysis of Epidemiologic Studies. Thyroid Research Journal. 9:1-9.

[29] Rivlin RS. Magnesium deficiency and alcohol intake: mechanisms, clinical significance and possible relation to cancer development (a review). J Am Coll Nutr 1994;13:416–23.

[30] Dean C. (2012 Jun 3). Magnesium – The Weight Loss Cure. Natural News. http://www.naturalnews.com/036049_magnesium_weight_loss_cure.html.

[31] Serefko A, Szopa A, Wlaź P, et al. (2013) Magnesium in depression. Pharmacological Reports. 65(3):547-54.

[32] Jacka FN, Overland S, Stewart R, et al. (2009 Jan) Association between magnesium intake and depression and anxiety in community-dwelling adults: the Hordaland Health Study. The Australian and New Zealand Journal of Psychiatry. 43(1):45-52. doi: 10.1080/00048670802534408.

[33] Shearer MJ. Role of vitamin K and Gla proteins in the pathophysiology of osteoporosis and vascular calcification. Current Opinion in Clinical Nutrition and Metabolic Care 2000; 3: 433–8.

[34] Szulc P, Arlot M, Chapuy MC, Duboeuf F, Meunier PJ, Delmas PD. Serum undercarboxylated osteocalcin correlates with hip bone mineral density in elderly women. Journal of Bone and Mineral Research 1994; 9: 1591–5.

[35] Knapen MH, Drummen NE, Smit E, Vermeer C, Theuwissen E. (2013 Sep 24). Three-year low-dose menaquinone-7 supplementation helps decrease bone loss in healthy postmenopausal women. *Osteoporosis International*. (9):2499–507.

[36] Beulens JW, Bots ML, Atsma F. Marie-Louise E.L. et al. (2008 Jul 07). High dietary menaquinone intake is associated with reduced coronary calcification. *Atherosclerosis*, 203, Issue 2, 489–493.

[37] Schurgers LJ, Cranenburg EC, Vermeer C. (2008 Sep 5). Matrix Gla-protein: the calcification inhibitor in need of vitamin K. *Thrombosis and Haemostasis*. 100(4):593-603. DOI: http://dx.doi.org/10.1160/TH08-02-0087.

[38] Marjo H. J. Knapen, Lavienja A. J. L. M. Braam, et al. (2015) Menaquinone-7 supplementation improves arterial stiffness in healthy postmenopausal women. Thrombosis and Haemostasis DOI: 10.1160/TH14-08-0675.

[39] Juanola-Falgarona M, Salas-Salvadó J, Martínez-González MÁ, et al. (2014 May). Dietary intake of vitamin K is inversely associated with mortality risk. The American Institute of Nutrition—Journal of Nutrition. 144(5):743-50.

[40] Yamaguchi M. (2010 May). Role of nutritional zinc in the prevention of osteoporosis. *Molecular and Cellular Biochemistry*. 338(1-2):241-54. doi: 10.1007/s11010-009-0358-0.

[41] Cilotti A, Falchetti A. Male osteoporosis and androgenic therapy: From testosterone to SARMs. Clin Cases Miner Bone Metab. 2009;6:229–33.

[42] Mohamad NV, Soelaiman IN, Chin KY. A concise review of testosterone and bone health. Clin Interv Aging. 2016;11:1317–24.

[43] Haase H, Rink L. (2009 June 12). The immune system and the impact of zinc during aging. *Immunity & Ageing*. 6: 9. doi: 10.1186/1742-4933-6-9.

[44] Singh RB, Niaz MA, Rastogi SS, Bajaj S, et al. (1998 Dec). Current zinc intake and risk of diabetes and coronary artery disease and factors associated with insulin resistance in rural and urban populations of *North India*. *Journal of the American College of Nutrition*. 17(6):564-70.

[45] Swardfager W. Ph.D , Herrmann N. M.D., Mazereeuw G. Ph.D Candidate, et al (2013 Dec 15). Zinc in Depression: A Meta-Analysis. *Biological Psychiatry*. 74, (12): 872–878.

[46] Payahoo L, Ostadrahimi A, Mobasseri M, et al. (2013). Effects of Zinc Supplementation on the Anthropometric Measurements, Lipid Profiles and Fasting Blood Glucose in the Healthy Obese Adults. *Advanced Pharmaceutical Bulletin*. 3(1), 161-165. doi: http://dx.doi.org/10.5681/apb.2013.027.

[47] Foster M, Chu A, Petocz P, Samman S. (2013 Aug 15). Effect of vegetarian diets on zinc status: a systematic review and meta-analysis of studies in humans. *Journal of the Science of Food and Agriculture*. 93(10):2362-71.

[48] Kim J. (2013 Dec). Dietary zinc intake is inversely associated with systolic blood pressure in young obese women. *Nutrition Research and Practice*. 7(6):519.

[49] Aranow C. (2011 Aug) Vitamin D and the Immune System. *J Investig Med*. 59(6): 881–886. doi: 10.231/JIM.0b013e31821b8755.

[50] Urashima M, Segawa T, Okazaki M, et al. (2010 May) Randomized trial of vitamin D supplementation to prevent seasonal influenza A in schoolchildren. *The American Journal of Clinical Nutrition*. 91(5):1255-60. doi: 10.3945/ajcn.2009.29094.

[51] Markose, Elizabeth R.; Stein, Janet L.; Stein, Gary S.; and Lian, Jane B., (1990 Mar) "Vitamin D-mediated modifications in protein-DNA interactions at two promoter elements of the osteocalcin gene."

[52] YoshihikoOhyamaToshimasaShinki (2015 Sep) Handbook of Hormones. Comparative Endocrinology for Basic and Clinical Research. Subchapter 97A–Calcitriol. https://doi.org/10.1016/B978-0-12-801028-0.00236-1.

[53] Pilz S1, Frisch S, Koertke H, Kuhn J, Dreier J, et al., (2011 Mar) Horm Metab Res. Effect of vitamin D supplementation on testosterone levels in men. doi: 10.1055/s-0030-1269854.

[54] John Cannell, MD (2012 Dec 28) Activated vitamin D vs 25(OH)D levels: What should you measure? Vitamin D Council.

[55] Rock CL, Emond JA, Flatt SW, et al. (2012 Nov). Weight loss is associated with increased serum 25-hydroxyvitamin D in overweight or obese women. *Obesity (Silver Spring, Md.)*. 20(11):2296-301.

[56] Schöttker B, Haug U, Schomburg L, et al. (2013 Apr) Strong associations of 25-hydroxyvitamin D concentrations with all-cause, cardiovascular, cancer, and respiratory disease mortality in a large cohort study. *Rev Med Interne.* 97(4):782-93. doi: 10.3945/ajcn.112.047712.

[57] Littlejohns T, Henley W, Lang IA, et al. (2014 Aug 6) Vitamin D and the risk of dementia and Alzheimer disease. *Neurology.* 29(10):815-20. doi: 10.1212/WNL.0000000000000755.

[58] 17. Preece M.A., Tomlinson S., Ribot C.A., Pietrek J., Korn H.T., Davies D.M. Studies of vitamin D deficiency in man. Q J Med. 1975;44:575–589.

[59] Dlugos D.J., Perrotta P.L., Horn W.G. Effects of the submarine environment on renal-stone risk factors and vitamin D metabolism. Undersea Hyperb Med. 1995;22:145–152.

[60] G. Haddad, John. (1992). Vitamin D — Solar Rays, the Milky Way, or Both?. New England journal of medicine. 326. 1213-5. 10.1056/NEJM199204303261808.

[61] "NIH Vitamin D Fact Sheet for Health Professionals," last reviewed June 24, 2011, http://ods.od.nih.gov/factsheets/VitaminD-HealthProfessional/.

[62] Mistretta VI, Delanaye P, Chapelle JP, et al. (2008 Oct) Vitamin D2 or vitamin D3. *Rev Med Interne.* 29(10):815-20. doi: 10.1016/j.revmed.2008.03.003.

[63] Houghton LA, Vieth R. (2006 Oct). The case against ergocalciferol (vitamin D2) as a vitamin supplement. *The American Journal of Clinical Nutrition.* 84(4):694-7.

[64] Independent (2017 March) https://www.independent.co.uk/news/uk/home-news/health-warning-over-toxic-levels-of-vitamin-d-sold-in-supplements-a7625331.html.

[65] Greene-Finestone L.S., Berger C., de Groh M., et al. 25-Hydroxyvitamin D in Canadian adults: biological, environmental, and behavioral correlates. Osteoporos Int. 2011;22:1389–1399.

[66] Mostafa WZ, Hegazy RA. Vitamin D and the skin: focus on a complex relationship: a review. J Adv Res. 2015;6(6):793–804. doi: 10.1016/j.jare.2014.01.011.

[67] "NIH Vitamin D Fact Sheet for Health Professionals," accessed July 24, 2014, http://ods.od.nih.gov/factsheets/VitaminD-HealthProfessional/.

[68] Kurt A. Kennel, MD, Matthew T. Drake, MD, PhD, and Daniel L. Hurley, MD (2010 Aug). Vitamin D Deficiency in Adults: When to Test and How to Treat 85(8): 752–758. doi: 10.4065/mcp.2010.0138.

[69] "NIH Vitamin D Fact Sheet for Health Professionals," accessed July 24, 2014, http://ods.od.nih.gov/factsheets/VitaminD-HealthProfessional/.

[70] Mostafa WZ, Hegazy RA. Vitamin D and the skin: focus on a complex relationship: a review. J Adv Res. 2015;6(6):793–804. doi: 10.1016/j.jare.2014.01.011.

[71] Vanchinathan V., Lim H.W. A dermatologist's perspective on vitamin D. Mayo Clin Proc. 2012;87:372–380.

[72] Holick MF, MacLaughlin JA, Doppelt SH. Regulation of cutaneous previtamin D3 photosynthesis in man: skin pigment is not an essential regulator. Science. 1981;211(4482):590-593.

[73] Victoria J. Drake, Ph.D., Daniel Bikle, M.D., Ph.D. (2011 Nov) Linus Pauling Institute: Micronutrient Information Center, Vitamin D and Skin Health. https://lpi.oregonstate.edu/mic/health-disease/skin-health/vitamin-D.

[74] Bruce W Hollis, Carol L Wagner; Assessment of dietary vitamin D requirements during pregnancy and lactation, The American Journal of Clinical Nutrition, Volume 79, Issue 5, 1 May 2004, Pages 717–726, https://doi.org/10.1093/ajcn/79.5.717

[75] Vitamin D Council (accessed Jan 22, 2019) Vitamin D and other vitamins and minerals https://www.vitamindcouncil.org/about-vitamin-d/vitamin-d-and-other-vitamins-and-minerals/#.XEbtXlVKjRY.

[76] "Testing for vitamin D," accessed July 16, 2014, http://www.vitamindcouncil.org/about-vitamin-d/testing-for-vitamin-d/.

[77] Nicole Cutler, L.Ac., MTCM, Dipl. Ac. (accessed Feb 1, 2019) Liver Health and Osteoporosis https://www.liversupport.com/improving-liver-disease-equals-improving-bone-health/.

[78] Navarro VJ, Barnhart H, Bonkovsky HL, et al. (2014) Liver injury from herbals and dietary supplements in the U.S. drug-induced liver injury network. Hepatology (2014) 60:1399–408. 10.1002/hep.27317

[79] Yu Zheng, Hong Zhou, James R.K. Modzelewski, et al. (2007 Oct) Accelerated Bone Resorption, Due to Dietary Calcium Deficiency, Promotes Breast Cancer Tumor Growth in Bone. American Association for Cancer Research (AACR).

[80] Salynn Boyles, Reviewed by Louise Chang, MD (2008 September 03) Calcium Levels Predict Prostate Cancer. https://www.webmd.com/prostate-cancer/news/20080903/calcium-levels-predict-prostate-cancer#1.

[81] "Magnesium and Heart Disease", accessed August 27, 2014, http://www.exatest.com/.

[82] "What Is a Coronary Calcium Scan?" accessed July 18, 2014, http://www.nhlbi.nih.gov/health/health-topics/topics/cscan/.

[83] WebMD Medical Reference Reviewed by James Beckerman, MD, FACC on July 6, 2018   What Is a Coronary Calcium Scan?

NOTES

[84] Calvo MS, Moshfegh AJ, Tucker KL. Assessing the health impact of phosphorus in the food supply: issues and considerations. Adv Nutr. 2014;5(1):104-113.

[85] Krajcovicová-Kudláčková M, Bucková K, Klimes I, et al (2003 Sep). Iodine Deficiency in Vegetarians and Vegans. *Nutrition & Metabolism.* (47):183–185.

[86] Delange F1, Bürgi H, Chen ZP, et al. (2002 Oct). World status of monitoring iodine deficiency disorders control programs. *Thyroid.* 12(10):915-24.

[87] "FAQs about Iodine Nutrition." Accessed September 3, 2014, http://www.iccidd.org/p142000264.html.

[88] "Iodine Deficiency", published June 4, 2012, http://www.thyroid.org/iodine-deficiency/.

[89] "ATA Statement on the Potential Risks of Excess Iodine Ingestion and Exposure," June 5, 2013, http://www.thyroid.org/ata-statement-on-the-potential-risks-of-excess-iodine-ingestion-and-exposure/.

[90] "Hashimoto's disease fact sheet", last updated July 16, 2012, http://womenshealth.gov/publications/our-publications/fact-sheet/hashimoto-disease.html.

[91] Weaver CM (2013 May) Potassium and health. 1;4(3):368S-77S. doi: 10.3945/an.112.003533.

[92] Elena Torreggiani, Annamaria Massa, Gemma Di Pompo1 et al. (2016) Bone Abstracts - The effect of potassium citrate on human primary osteoclasts in vitro 5 P202 | DOI: 10.1530/boneabs.5.P202.

[93] Megan Ware RDN LD. (2018, January 10). "Everything you need to know about potassium." Medical News Today. Retrieved from https://www.medicalnewstoday.com/articles/287212.php.

[94] Rude RK, Shils ME., Shike M, et al. (2006) Modern Nutrition in Health and Disease. 10th ed. *Lippincott Williams & Wilkins*, 2006:223-247.

[95] "Multivitamin/mineral Supplements Fact Sheet for Health Professionals," last reviewed Jan 07, 2013, http://ods.od.nih.gov/factsheets/MVMS-HealthProfessional/.

[96] Guallar E, Stranges S, Mulrow C, et al. (2013 Dec 17) Enough Is Enough: Stop Wasting Money on Vitamin and Mineral Supplements. *Annals of Internal Medicine.* 159(12):850-851. doi:10.7326/0003-4819-159-12-201312170-00011.

[97] "A daily multivitamin is a great nutrition insurance policy," accessed July 27, 2014, http://www.hsph.harvard.edu/nutritionsource/what-should-you-eat/vitamins/.

[98] Huang HY, Caballero B, Chang S, et al. (2006 May) The Efficacy and Safety of Multivitamin and Mineral Supplement Use to Prevent Cancer and Chronic Disease in Adults: A Systematic Review for a NIH State-of-the-Science Conference. *Annals of Internal Medicine*, 145:372-385.

NOTES

99 Criteria used to compare multivitamin brands can be found at: http://www.multivitaminguide.org/study-methodology.html.

100 Mowe M, Bohmer T, Kindt E. (1994) Reduced nutritional status in an elderly population (.70 year) is probable before disease and possibly contributes to the development of disease. *American Journal of Clinical Nutrition*

101 Larsson J, Unosson M, Ek A-C, Nilsson L, et al. Effect of dietary supplement on nutritional status and clinical outcome in 501 geriatric patients—a randomised study. *Clinical Nutrition* 1990; 9: 179–84.

102 Pan A, Sun Q, Bernstein AM, et al. (2011 April 9) Red meat consumption and mortality: results from 2 prospective cohort studies. *Archives of Internal Medicine*. 172(7):555-63. doi: 10.1001/archinternmed.2011.2287.

103 Jeukendrup AE. (2010 Jul). Carbohydrate and exercise performance: the role of multiple transportable carbohydrates. *Current Opinion in Clinical Nutrition and Metabolic Care*. 13(4):452-7. doi: 10.1097/MCO.0b013e328339de9f.

104 Yen CM, Kuo CL, Lin MC, et al. (2014 Nov) Sleep disorders increase the risk of osteoporosis: a nationwide population-based cohort study. *Sleep Medicine* 15.11 (2014): 1339-1344. doi: 10.1016/j.sleep.2014.07.005.

105 Cunningham TD, Di Pace BS. (2015 Jul) Is Self-Reported Sleep Duration Associated with Osteoporosis? Data from a 4-Year Aggregated Analysis from the National Health and Nutrition Examination Survey. *Journal of American Geriatrics Society*. 63.7 (2015): 1401-1406.

106 Xiaowen X, Liang W, Liying C, et al. (2016 Aug) Effects of chronic sleep deprivation on bone mass and bone metabolism in rats. *Journal of Orthopaedic Surgery and Research*. doi: 10.1186/s13018-016-0418-6

107 Hublin C, Partinen M, Koskenvuo M, et al. (2007) Sleep and mortality: a population-based 22-year follow-up study. *Sleep*. 30(10):1245-1253.

108 CDC. (2013 Jul 1). Sleep and Sleep Disorders. CDC, National Center for Chronic Disease Prevention and Health Promotion, Division of Population Health. http://www.cdc.gov/sleep/.

109 Pablos MI, Agapito MT, Gutierrez-Baraja R, et al (1996 Oct) Effect of calcium on melatonin secretion in chick pineal gland I. *Elsevier Science Direct*. 18;217(2-3):161-4. doi.org/10.1016/0304-3940(96)13101-3.

110 Gulseren Akyuz, Moira O'Brien, Mehrsheed Sinaki, et al., (accessed 2019 Feb) Exercise Recommendations. *International Osteoporosis Foundation*.

111 "Supplement", accessed Jul 25, 2014, http://www.merriam-webster.com/dictionary/supplement

112 9.Murray CW, Egan SK, Kim H, et al. (2008 Nov) US Food and Drug Administration's Total Diet Study: dietary intake of perchlorate and iodine. *J Expo Sci Environ Epidemiol*. 18(6):571-580. doi: 10.1038/sj.jes.7500648.

Made in United States
Troutdale, OR
12/29/2024

27390451R00100